Using the
GAPS DIET

175 Recipes for Gaining Control of Your Gut Flora

Signe Gad

Introduction by Dr. Irene Hage, MD, ND

For complete cataloguing information, see page 279.

Disclaimer

This book is a general guide only and should never be a substitute for the skill, knowledge and experience of a qualified medical professional dealing with the facts, circumstances and symptoms of a particular case.

The nutritional, medical and health information presented in this book is based on the research, training and professional experience of the author, and is true and complete to the best of her knowledge. However, this book is intended only as an informative guide for those wishing to know more about health, nutrition and medicine; it is not intended to replace or countermand the advice given by the reader's personal physician. Because each person and situation is unique, the author and the publisher urge the reader to check with a qualified health-care professional before using any procedure where there is a question as to its appropriateness. The author and the publisher are not responsible for any adverse effects or consequences resulting from the use of the information in this book. It is the responsibility of the reader to consult a physician or other qualified health-care professional regarding their personal care.

This book contains references to products that may not be available everywhere. The intent of the information provided is to be helpful; however, there is no guarantee of results associated with the information provided. Use of brand names is for educational purposes only and does not imply endorsement.

The recipes in this book have been carefully tested by our kitchen and our tasters. To the best of our knowledge, they are safe and nutritious for ordinary use and users. For those people with food or other allergies, or who have special food requirements or health issues, please read the suggested contents of each recipe carefully and determine whether or not they may create a problem for you. All recipes are used at the risk of the consumer. We cannot be responsible for any hazards, loss or damage that may occur as a result of any recipe use. For those with special needs, allergies, requirements or health problems, in the event of any doubt, please contact your medical adviser prior to the use of any recipe.

Design and production: Daniella Zanchetta/PageWave Graphics Inc.
Translator: Nina Sokol
Proofreader: Kelly Jones
Indexer: Gillian Watts

Cover image: Ingredients on slate background © Phive2015/iStock/Getty Images Plus
Back cover images: Bowl of broth © iStock.com/margouillatphotos; Slate background © iStock.com/themacx

Published by Robert Rose Inc.
120 Eglinton Avenue East, Suite 800, Toronto, Ontario, Canada M4P 1E2
Tel: (416) 322-6552 Fax: (416) 322-6936
www.robertrose.ca

Printed and bound in Canada

1 2 3 4 5 6 7 8 9 MI 26 25 24 23 22 21 20 19 18

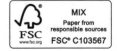

Contents

Foreword

I would like to thank Signe Gad for writing this cookbook! GAPS stands for "gut and psychology syndrome" or "gut and physiology syndrome," and it includes all of the health problems that stem from unhealthy gut flora. The gut flora is a large community of microbes that live inside the human digestive system. Research has shown that it consists of 10 times as many cells as does the human body itself. So our bodies are only 10% of us; the body is a shell and a habitat for the mass of microbes that live inside us. We ignore them at our peril, because they fulfill a myriad of functions in the human body. Your digestion, your stamina, your strength, your immune function, your ability to cope with daily stress and pressure, and even your thoughts and emotions are dependent on the health of your gut flora.

Our modern environment is filled with influences that damage people's gut flora on an unprecedented level. Our food and water are full of chemicals and antibiotics that kill certain microbes in the gut, leaving other microbes out of balance. We take pharmaceutical medications, which alter the composition of our gut flora. The majority of people in the Western world have damaged gut flora and, as a result, are not healthy. The first part of the body to suffer from this damage is the digestive system. In this book, Signe Gad describes her daughter's digestive illness very well, and how her daughter has recovered.

About 85% of our immune system is located in the gut wall. When the gut flora is abnormal, the immune system becomes ill and we develop allergies and autoimmune disease (rheumatoid arthritis, multiple sclerosis, type 1 diabetes, lupus, etc.). An unhealthy gut flora damages the gut wall, making it porous and leaky. As a result, a river of toxins and undigested food flows into the bloodstream, overwhelming the liver and other detoxification organs. People in this situation develop food allergies and food intolerances, chronic fatigue syndrome, fibromyalgia and other debilitating conditions.

The gut flora is a large community of microbes that live inside the human digestive system. Recent research has discovered that there are ten times as many microbes in our gut flora as in the rest of our bodies!

When this river of toxicity gets to the brain, the person develops mental illness: depression, obsessive-compulsive disorder, bipolar disorder, schizophrenia, eating disorders, addictions, etc. If this situation happens in a baby or a small child, the child may develop autism, ADHD, dyslexia, dyspraxia or other learning disabilities.

All of these conditions are GAPS. The good news is that we can heal our gut flora and our gut wall. Once they are healed and the gut flora becomes healthy and normal, all of the other GAPS-related illnesses in the body start disappearing. The GAPS nutritional protocol has been designed to do that. It is described in detail in my book *Gut and Psychology Syndrome: Natural Treatment for Autism, Dyslexia, ADHD, Dyspraxia, Depression and More*.

This cookbook will give you guidelines on how to heal using the GAPS diet. It has delicious healthy recipes to follow, and good information about the gut flora and its role in human health. I applaud Signe Gad for writing this book and warmly recommend it!

— *Natasha Campbell-McBride, MD*
June 2016

About 85% of our immune system is located in the gut wall. When the gut flora is abnormal, the immune system becomes ill and we develop allergies and autoimmune disease.

For Karen

Preface: Karen's Story

Although I am not a chef, nutritional expert or practitioner of any kind, I managed to help my daughter, Karen, get rid of her chronic stomachaches, from which she had been suffering for over 7 years, since the age of 4. Our "rounds of practitioners" — which included both established and alternative practitioners — did not end until we landed with a functional medical practitioner, Dr. Irene Hage, who mentioned the word "GAPS." Once I did some research on GAPS, I took it from there, because I had learned that it would be a battle fought mostly in the kitchen.

It would later become evident that following the GAPS diet meant putting in several years of focused effort before Karen would be able to have a life where she wasn't tormented by constant stomachaches. When we plunged into the diet, there were neither professional nor experienced GAPS practitioners in Denmark, where we live, much less information on GAPS in Danish. The mere idea of familiarizing myself with the complexity of problems associated with GAPS was a time-consuming endeavor, but it made so much sense to me that I was close to getting on a soapbox in the middle of Copenhagen's town square to shout my message to the world.

And then there was the practical aspect of it all. I definitely could have used a good cookbook, so that I wouldn't have had to reinvent the wheel on a daily basis.

Some of the questions I had, for example, were:

- How do I actually get started?
- What can I put in my daughter's lunch bag when I cannot make sandwiches?
- How do you get baked goods to taste good when you cannot use starch, sugar, yeast or baking powder?
- How do you make GAPS food for a whole week when your child is going away to camp?
- What do you do when all of her friends, with the best of intentions, offer her candy, cakes, bread and pasta?
- How do you generally handle events and trips abroad?

The point of departure for these questions is, logically enough, based on what you *cannot* eat when you are on a GAPS diet. So you might be thinking, "Oh no, not another one of those horrible diets that requires you to exclude all kinds of food."

I managed to help my daughter, Karen, get rid of her chronic stomachaches, from which she had been suffering for over 7 years.

Although it is true that you have to give up sugar, starch and processed food, including additives, while on the GAPS diet, I also quickly learned that:

- The GAPS diet focuses mainly on not only what you *can* eat, but on what you *should* eat. That is why I call it a "yes" diet, unlike most other diets that, because of their focus on numerous restrictions, are "no" diets.

- The GAPS diet gives you the opportunity to experiment with tasty, high-quality food, which is to say homemade meals made from food products of excellent quality. (I say homemade because that way you know what the food contains. But if you can get others to make food of the same quality, then it doesn't necessarily have to be made at home!)

- Following the GAPS diet is basically just a matter of thinking and prioritizing differently than you are used to.

- The GAPS diet has nothing to do with being on a low-fat vegetarian diet, or with counting calories.

- The GAPS diet is not a healthy-within-such-and-such-a-brief-period-of-time type of diet. Healing takes time, especially when it comes to changing the condition of your internal biochemistry.

I baked nut muffins with berries for when the others got cupcakes, and gave her apple cider when there was a chance that juice or soda might be served.

How did things go with Karen? Once she started following the GAPS diet, the constant bloating she was suffering from disappeared after a week, and the stomachaches slowly disappeared as well. For an 11-year-old, she was impressively good at sticking to the diet. She understood and believed that her persistence would contribute to sending her terrible pain to Timbuktu. But I was also good at helping her. I prioritized cooking at home and spent considerably longer in the kitchen than I normally would have.

I always made sure that Karen had her own alternative to sugary and starchy foods whenever she went out. For example, she always had a fruit-cocoa bar in her schoolbag to eat when the other children got snacks at school — the kind that has no added sugar, not even the new fancy types like processed stevia or palm sugar. Although she liked these bars, they weren't exactly her favorite thing. But once she got through a 16-day period of going cold turkey on sugar, her interest in sugar declined considerably.

I baked nut muffins with berries for when the others got cupcakes, and gave her apple cider when there was a chance that juice or soda might be served. I managed to conjure up GAPS sushi when Karen announced that she and her friends had planned a sushi party. By sheer luck, I had some gravlax in the fridge that I could use.

In general, I made sure to have a vast array of food products stored in the freezer, fridge and pantry at all times, and I was always planning for the near future when it came to meals and snacks.

This amount of work may sound mind-boggling and completely overwhelming. Yes, you have to be prepared for extra effort in the beginning, until new routines become new habits. The brain is lazy by nature, so you have to use it consciously when you are doing something different than you are used to. This new diet demands attention, pure and simple. It also requires that you make an effort to turn your head in new directions when grocery shopping, and that you do a little more research to find tools or food products that are new to you. You must also think a few days ahead and make it a routine to start preparing new portions before the last ones are consumed. Any sourdough baker can tell you all about that, since sourdough bread takes a few days to make. It's not worse than that.

I learned to tackle the new cuisine by taking one step at a time over a long period. After a while, I also learned the importance of thorough and clear communication with friends, family and other adults who deal with your child on a daily basis. We were lucky enough to have friends who were considerate and served up the most delicious GAPS-oriented meals — which they themselves enjoyed eating. But there were, on occasion, situations that Karen, as an 11-year-old, could have done without, such as when, on an outing, a teacher from another school announced, "Hey, right now we're cooking for the group (spaghetti with meat sauce), so you'll just have to wait to make your own food." Fortunately, a teacher from our school, whom I had informed about Karen's diet, came to her rescue after a little while.

Karen continued the diet for exactly 2 years and is now able to eat starch and sugar in limited quantities. I repeat: limited! She still needs proper food — that is, as few processed ingredients as possible. She has learned from bitter experience that a week of junk food and sloppy meal habits creates the potential for relapse. For the rest of her life, she will have to really think about what she eats and eat properly, but she can afford to go berserk every now and then without getting sick. There is no need for her to repeatedly go on a restrictive diet to keep the symptoms at bay; she can simply relax and concentrate on living her life.

— *Signe Gad*
September 2017

> *In general, I made sure to have a vast array of food products stored in the freezer, fridge and pantry at all times, and I was always planning for the near future when it came to meals and snacks.*

Introduction

My thanks to Signe Gad, who has written this wonderful book and created healthy, healing GAPS recipes that are easy, fun and taste fantastic!

Signe came into my office several years ago with her daughter, Karen, then 11 years old. From a very young age, Karen had suffered from quite severe abdominal pain and cramps. No explanation could be found, and no treatments helped. Signe and Karen were told over and over again that "Children get stomachaches — it's normal." But these were more than just "wanting to stay home" kind of stomachaches.

After hearing Karen's medical history, I suspected that she had gut dysbiosis (unbalanced gut microorganisms) and a gut lining issue (leaky gut). Bowel tests confirmed the diagnosis, and I recommended what I saw as the most thorough and well-investigated diet for healing the gut: the GAPS diet.

Signe dived into reading and got to know everything about the GAPS diet. I admired her commitment. Because she already had a background as a holistic body worker and had been raised in a family of respected doctors, I knew she would understand the use and full significance of the GAPS diet. Thanks to Signe's diligence, Karen improved remarkably within a few months and today is an active and happy young woman.

As a medical doctor with a keen interest in holistic naturopathic medicine, I have come across numerous patients with chronic symptoms that cannot be explained, symptoms ranging from fatigue, headaches and brain fog to bowel issues, obesity, muscle weakness and many more. Their test results are normal, and they are often told that their problem must be genetic or stress-related.

In my 28 years of medical experience, I have observed that, where no other causative factor can be determined, symptoms and health conditions often originate in the gut. Hippocrates' maxim "Let food be thy medicine" rings truer than ever — but what and how should we be eating, and why?

As we hear so often, more and more people are contracting and dying from cancer, diabetes, heart and lung diseases, but less commonly reported is that once-rare conditions — such as autoimmune diseases, dementia, adrenal burnout, thyroid conditions, attention deficit hyperactivity disorder (ADHD), depression and autism — are steeply on the rise.

As the incidence of chronic diseases increases, we are becoming more and more aware of the importance of diet,

As a medical doctor, I have come across numerous patients with chronic symptoms that cannot be explained, symptoms ranging from fatigue, headaches and brain fog to bowel issues, obesity, muscle weakness and many more. I have observed that, where no other causative factor can be determined, symptoms and health conditions often originate in the gut.

elimination of toxins through lifestyle changes, a healthy digestive system and a healthy immune system. According to the U.S. Centers for Disease Control and Prevention (CDC), eliminating poor diet, inactivity and smoking would prevent 80% of all heart disease and stroke, 80% of type 2 diabetes and 40% of cancers.

Closely related to our diet and digestion is the microbiome — the body's array of bacteria and other microorganisms. An increasing amount of research points to the importance of the composition of these microorganisms within the body. There are beneficial microorganisms, and there are pathogenic (disease-causing) microorganisms. The gut microbiome is like a separate organ of its own, and it is affected by diet, physical activity, antibiotics, prebiotics, hormones, stress, living with animals and heavy metals. The microorganisms in our gut play a huge role in our health, from prevention of disease to what type of illness we may get — all dependent on which microorganisms we carry, and in what quantity.

Dr. Natasha Campbell-McBride has shown through extensive research that many chronic conditions, such as leaky gut (in which the gut lining is damaged) and dysbiosis (unhealthy microorganisms in the gut), are associated with intestinal issues. She coined the term "gut and psychology syndrome (GAPS)," which establishes the connection between the digestive system and the neurological system. Through her guidance, many people have been able to address the root cause of their chronic conditions, and by following the GAPS diet have been able to heal their bodies. (For more information, visit www.gaps.me.)

Using the GAPS Diet provides a good overview of how one can become ill because of poor gut function. After reading the first part of the book, you will be well informed about GAPS and will be able to start following the principles of the GAPS diet and begin the healing process. Thankfully, Signe also brings the GAPS diet to a new gastronomic level, where the taste, texture, and appearance of the food are just as important as in any other collection of mouthwatering recipes.

I have many patients with a chronic condition who need a gut-friendly, healing, tasty and fulfilling diet. I am grateful that Signe has created and tested so many wonderful recipes and written this cookbook. It offers numerous meals and ideas for the many people who may find it difficult to get started or just want something straightforward and simple to prepare.

I know the book you hold will be a great support in your daily home cooking while you are on a GAPS diet.

— *Irene Hage, MD, ND*
September 2017

The microorganisms in our gut play a huge role in our health, from prevention of disease to what type of illness we may get — all dependent on which microorganisms we carry, and in what quantity.

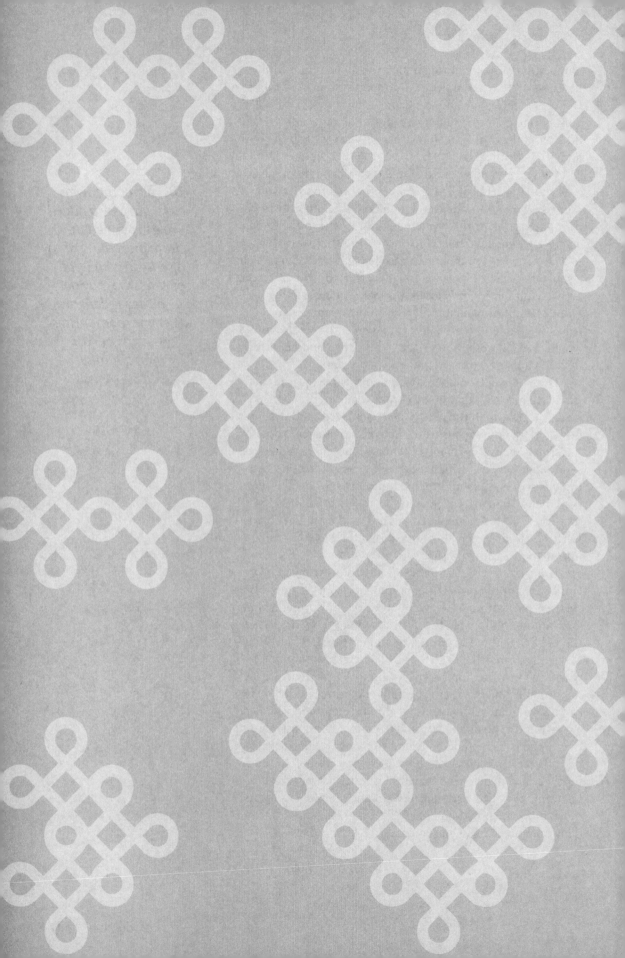

PART 1

Getting Started with the GAPS Diet

What Is GAPS?

Gut and psychology syndrome — or GAPS — is a generic term used for a range of modern chronic diseases that all derive from compromised intestinal flora. The diagnosis was introduced in 2004 by neurologist and nutritional expert Natasha Campbell-McBride, whose son had a past diagnosis related to autism. Dr. Campbell-McBride is a pioneer when it comes to explaining the connection between our health and the state of our intestinal flora, and she has developed a natural and medication-free solution for people suffering from GAPS-related chronic diagnoses or symptoms: the GAPS diet.

In recent years, gut microbiota have become a hot topic for researchers the world over. The influx of research findings on the subject has intensified and further substantiated what we "Gapsters" — those of us who are following or have followed the GAPS diet — have already discovered in real life: that our physical and mental well-being depend to a large extent on the condition of our intestinal flora.

Crash Course in the Gut Flora

Digestion is a complicated business. The intestine lacks oxygen, so it is difficult to recreate the same environment with the same microbes in a research laboratory. As a result, the knowledge we have been able to gain based on solid, reliable research has been limited. Fortunately, research methods are constantly improving.

Here's what we do know, based on both research and the consistent experiences of many people living in the real world: to be in good health, our intestines must contain hundreds of species and subspecies of bacteria and other microbes. An adult human's gut contains about 4.4 pounds (2 kg) of these microbes, which can be divided into three groups:

- **Beneficial microbes** (also called "probiotics") provide numerous health benefits.
- **Opportunistic microbes** assist the beneficial bacteria in a healthy gut, but can turn on a dime in a disrupted gut flora, taking advantage of the opportunity to become harmful bacteria instead.
- **Harmful microbes** damage our health, leading to various illnesses and diseases.

Did You Know?

Microbiota = Gut Flora

For practical reasons, it may be useful to know that another term for the gut flora, used mainly by scholars, is "microbiota." I tend to use the term "gut flora," because it's a more colorful, less clinical term that is better suited for everyday language.

Ideally, beneficial bacteria would dominate the environment of the gut, with harmful bacteria absent or minimal. Although harmful bacteria are constantly making their way into the body, beneficial bacteria make sure that they are quickly expelled. That is why harmful bacteria are also called "transitional" bacteria — in a healthy, well-functioning gut, they don't stick around for long.

Beneficial microbes, assisted by opportunistic microbes, have many different functions that keep you healthy, happy and, quite simply, alive! In addition to weeding out harmful bacteria, they oversee the maintenance of the digestive system in collaboration with enzymes, vitamins and minerals (among others) and help you absorb vital nutrients. They play a role in the immune system, in hormone production, in metabolism and in cell function, contributing to your energy levels, your resistance to physical and mental illnesses, your sleep quality and your brain function.

The key to a well-functioning gut is diversity: the more types of beneficial and opportunistic microspecies that are present, the better. When the number and variety of beneficial species diminish, the intestinal environment's defenses become weakened, allowing not only health-damaging bacteria but also parasites and other unwanted microbes to enter freely and settle down.

As if that weren't enough, as the beneficial species decline, the opportunistic species take the opportunity to spread, taking advantage of their altered environment to become harmful instead of supportive. An example of this phenomenon is the opportunistic fungus *Candida albicans*, which, if it isn't held at bay by beneficial "microbe colleagues," spreads out of control, resulting in unpleasant and exhausting symptoms, such as bloating.

Did You Know?

About the Immune System

Seventy-five to 85% of the body's immune system is found inside the intestinal wall. So it's not surprising that one of the joyous results of healing your gut is that your immune system gains strength.

Sugar and Starch Feed Harmful Microbes

A Gapster's digestive system is in no condition to digest sugar and starch. Sugar is a disaccharide — a carbohydrate that consists of two connected molecules. Starch, which is found in foods such as potatoes, corn and grains, is a polysaccharide: a carbohydrate that consists of chains of many connected molecules. Since the body can absorb only one molecule at a time, connected molecules must first be split apart before they can be digested. A well-functioning intestine is able to do this. But a poorly functioning intestine, where the hierarchy has been upset, is unable to split the connected molecules, and instead of being digested, they become food for harmful bacteria, fungi and parasites. (If you would like to learn more about this issue, the reference list on page 276 includes resources that offer a thorough explanation of the problem.)

For that reason, sugar and all forms of starch are excluded from the GAPS diet — damaging microbes should not be fed! That doesn't mean you can never eat anything sweet: you can use honey or ripe fruit as sweeteners. There are plenty of dessert recipes in this book; they are simply made without sugar or flour.

In other words, the many trillions of bacteria and other microbes in the intestine live in a harmonious hierarchy. But if the number and variety of species shrink, the hierarchy is disturbed and a healthy gut flora transforms into one that is functioning poorly, initiating a number of chain reactions that result in various symptoms, ranging from mild to severe.

Leaky Gut Syndrome

The long-term presence of both harmful bacteria and sugar in the gut causes the intestinal wall to become porous and full of holes, a condition known as leaky gut syndrome. A leaky gut compromises the immune system, much of which is located inside the intestinal wall. The tightly knit barrier between the intestine and the bloodstream becomes a sieve through which toxic substances enter the bloodstream and can affect the brain, which can result in numerous mental and behavioral problems.

Furthermore, various food elements may seep out through the leaky intestinal wall, which may trigger the body's defense cells to form antibodies to combat the alien substances in the bloodstream. As a result, food allergies and intolerances are a classic GAPS symptom (although GAPS may not be the only cause of allergies). For more information on food allergies and intolerances, see page 42.

Did You Know?

GAPS Commonalities

Gapsters typically have several symptoms, not just one, and GAPS-related symptoms and diagnoses tend to run in families. Once Gapsters begin to follow the GAPS diet, their mental imbalances, if any, are the first to disappear, followed by their physical symptoms.

GAPS-Related Symptoms and Diagnoses

The number of GAPS-related symptoms and diagnoses continues to grow. To see an updated list, visit www.gaps.me. Below is a selection of some common symptoms and diagnoses. Please bear in mind that no one doubts the fact that there may be other causes than GAPS for the diagnoses mentioned here.

A	acid reflux (heartburn), acne, alcoholism, allergies, anorexia, anxiety, arrhythmia, arthritis, asthma, attention deficit hyperactivity disorder (ADHD), autism spectrum disorders, autoimmune reactions
B	back pains, bags under the eyes, bed-wetting, behavioral problems, bipolar disorder, bladder infection, bloating, blood pressure problems (high or low), bulimia
C	*Candida albicans* overgrowth, catarrh (esophageal, gastric), chronic cough, chronic inflammation*, circulatory problems, colic, concentration issues (difficulty concentrating), constipation, Crohn's disease
D	depression, diabetes (types 1 and 2), diarrhea, digestive problems, dizziness, dyslexia, dyspraxia
E	ear infections, eating disorders, eczema, epilepsy, esophageal hernia
F	fastidiousness, fibromyalgia, food allergies and intolerances
G	gout, growth problems, gum disease
H	hair loss, hardening of the arteries, hay fever, headaches, heart problems, hemorrhoids, high blood pressure, high sensitivity, histamine intolerance, hives (urticaria), hormonal problems
I	immune system dysfunction, infertility, intestinal infections, iron deficiency, irritable bowel syndrome (IBS)
K	kidney problems
L	learning disabilities, low blood pressure, lung infection, lupus
M	memory issues, menstruation problems, migraines, mood swings, multiple sclerosis, muscle spasms in legs, myalgic encephalomyelitis
N	narcolepsy, nausea, neurological problems, nightmares
O	obesity, obsessive compulsive disorder (OCD), overweight
P	parasites, plantar fasciitis, premenstrual syndrome (PMS), psoriasis, psychosis
R	receding gums, rosacea
S	schizophrenia, sinusitis, skin dryness, sleeping problems, stomachaches, stuffy nose, stuttering, sugar dependency
T	throat infections (recurrent), thyroid problems, tics, tooth discoloration, tooth sensitivity
U	ulcerative colitis, underweight, unstable blood sugar
V	vision problems, vomiting

Chronic inflammation is triggered by, among other things, harmful chemicals that may be present in our environment, in food we ingest, in products we use on our skin and in intestinal microbes.

The Purpose of the GAPS Diet

Did You Know?

A "Real Food" Diet

It may sound like I am about to begin a lecture promoting starvation diets and fat-free vegetarian food. I'm not! What the GAPS diet encourages you to eat, and what I will recommend throughout this book, is real food, the kind that is homemade from healthful ingredients that are varied, tasty, satisfying and full of nutrition for you and your loved ones.

Eating fermented foods every day, and preferably with each meal, is a firmly entrenched part of the diet.

If you find yourself with GAPS symptoms, you can take comfort in the fact that your inner biochemical condition is not a fixed entity. It can be adjusted, and that is exactly what the GAPS diet aims to do: to adjust your diet so that it detoxifies, restores, nourishes and becomes balanced.

Healing your gut is not going to happen overnight, and the GAPS diet is not a quick fix: it can take 2 years or more to progress through the diet and see full relief from your symptoms. So it's important to understand the thinking behind the diet so that you don't end up losing patience with it. With that in mind, these are the changes you are aiming for while following the GAPS diet:

1. **To rebuild your intestinal wall:** Your leaky intestinal wall must be patched up, which you can do with the help of certain kinds of foods, particularly slow-cooked bone broth. Learn more about bone broth and stock on page 98, and look for recipes on pages 99–103.

2. **To achieve a balanced gut flora:** Out with the bad and in with the good! This means eliminating damaging substances from the body to detoxify it, while eating foods that encourage the growth of beneficial bacteria. Vegetables — and, in particular, freshly pressed vegetable juices — help with detoxification, and fermented foods are an indispensable source of beneficial bacteria and fungi species. Eating fermented foods every day, and preferably with each meal, is a firmly entrenched part of the diet. For more information on freshly pressed juices, see the box on page 204. For more information on fermented foods, see pages 82 and 90.

3. **To build up your ability to absorb nutrients:** A toxic gut flora creates havoc in our complicated metabolism, and the body's ability to absorb vital nutrients becomes weakened. The GAPS diet is designed to remedy this, through the consumption of fats that benefit your health: saturated fats (including animal fats and coconut oil) and cold-pressed monounsaturated fats such as olive oil. Saturated fats? Yes, you read that correctly. For more on why saturated fats are an important part of the GAPS diet, see page 39. And you can learn more about the different types of fat and how to use them in the chapter "The Skinny on Fat," on page 36.

Through these measures to heal your gut, the long-term purposes of the GAPS diet are:

- to get rid of or minimize your GAPS-related symptoms and diagnoses;
- to allow you to once again consume fat, protein and carbohydrates in all their natural forms;
- to keep your symptoms at bay without you having to return to a restrictive diet at regular intervals.

These achievements are possible for most people who have been through the healing process of the GAPS diet, but there is one condition: that after the diet and for the rest of your life, you make sure to eat real food made with good-quality, unprocessed ingredients. You will most likely be able to tolerate starches such as rice and potatoes by the end of the diet. That goes for bread, too, but as always, choose well: in this case, your best option is sourdough bread made from good-quality whole-grain flour (a couple of bread recipes appear near the end of the book, on pages 273 and 274). You may be able to tolerate small amounts of sugar as an ingredient in healthy meals and baked goods, but if you're not making your own treats, make sure to select products that have been processed as little as possible.

> ## Did You Know?
>
> **Detoxification**
> Freshly pressed vegetable juices are great for detoxification, but you can also use other cleansing methods during the diet. A GAPS practitioner (see page 48) can guide you in safe detoxification practices.

What to Eat on the GAPS Diet

The GAPS diet is divided into three parts:

- The intro diet
- The full GAPS diet
- The transition diet

The intro diet has the most food exclusions, to provide a period of intense healing for your gut as you move through its six stages, gradually adding foods back into your diet one at a time. On the full diet, you have a lot more choice, although you will still want to introduce new foods gradually until you are sure you can tolerate them.

You will stay on the GAPS diet until your gut is fully healed and you are symptom-free, typically $1\frac{1}{2}$ to 2 years, but depending on diagnosis, some people need up to 5 years — this is not a quick fix! When you have been free of symptoms for 6 months, you will be ready for the transition diet, during which you can start to eat more starchy foods, such as new potatoes and sourdough bread baked with good-quality flour, and gradually add in whole grains (so long as you don't experience any setbacks!).

The Intro Diet

The intro diet in its entirety is intended to last for 3 to 6 weeks, but the time needed varies from person to person. People with severe GAPS may need to follow the intro diet for many months, or perhaps even for more than a year.

This part of the diet is the most stringent and starts with a limited selection of foods, which you can eat as much of and as often as you like. As you progress through the six stages of the intro diet (and presumably begin to feel better), you will start to include more and more foods.

The stages are designed to make the intro diet more systematic and manageable. It may sound complicated, but it isn't; on the contrary, the division into stages is a great help. You simply go through the stages, step by step, at whatever pace you need.

The purposes of the intro diet are:

- to rev up the healing of your intestinal wall through the consumption of homemade stock;
- to kick-start the detoxification process by, among other things, avoiding dietary fiber, drinking freshly pressed vegetable juices and consuming probiotics; and
- to clearly establish whether there are any foods you cannot tolerate.

By starting with a very restricted diet and adding foods back in one at a time, you become more sensitive and thereby better able to register whether a particular food makes you unwell. You may even discover that your discomfort is connected to something you did not realize was a problem. As the diet progresses, you may tolerate certain foods again; it varies from person to person. For example, you might learn that you can tolerate egg yolks but not egg whites, though you previously believed that eggs in general were an issue for you.

The stages are designed to make the intro diet more systematic and manageable. It may sound complicated, but it isn't; on the contrary, the division into stages is a great help.

Did You Know?

When and How to Use the Intro Diet

You don't necessarily need to start with the intro diet. Complete it when you are ready. Many people jump right into the full GAPS diet and work their way through the intro diet later. You can also repeat the intro diet whenever it suits you. A deeper and faster healing process takes place during the intro diet. Gapsters recount how they have managed to take an even bigger leap up the health ladder each time they have repeated it.

What to Eat on the Intro Diet

On the following pages, you will find lists of what you can eat at each stage of the intro diet. At a minimum, you should spend 3 days in each stage, but bear in mind that the amount of time you need to spend in each stage is extremely individual. Discuss your needs with your GAPS practitioner (see page 48), who can guide you through the intro diet so that it is customized just for you.

As you add foods back into your diet, one by one, take note of any food you are having trouble tolerating and what symptoms you experienced as a result. Keep detailed written notes so you can remember your experiences when you want to give that food another go. Wait a while before trying it again.

If you suspect that you might have a true food allergy, rather than an intolerance caused by a leaky gut, take the sensitivity test below *before* ingesting the food.

How to Test Your Sensitivity to Food Products

If you want to find out whether you can tolerate a food (for example, whey from your homemade yogurt) without eating it, dab a little bit on the inside of your wrist, where the skin is thin, right before going to bed. You can mash non-fluid foods in a little water. If an angry red rash appears on that spot by the next morning, then you cannot tolerate that food and are most likely allergic to it. If you do not have a reaction, you can most likely tolerate it — if not right away, then later, as you progress through the diet. Eat a tiny bit to begin with and wait a day or 3 before attempting to increase your intake.

Stage 1

- Meat stock based on at least 80% meat, made with parts including marrow, gelatin and connective tissue, boiled for $1\frac{1}{2}$ to 2 hours (you can also eat the meats, including the natural fats, marrow and tissue, that you strain out of the stock)

- Fish stock based on at least 80% fish, boiled for $1\frac{1}{2}$ hours

- Soups based on meat or fish stock that meet all other criteria for stage 1

- Vegetables without coarse fiber, boiled until very tender: bell peppers, carrots, cauliflower florets (without stems), celery root, green beans, green peas, leeks, mushrooms, onions, pumpkin, spinach, squash, zucchini; other boiled vegetables that do not contain too much fiber can also be used, but be sure to remove any coarse stems
- Garlic
- Ginger, with a little honey (optional)
- Peppercorns (all colors)
- Sauerkraut brine
- Whey from homemade yogurt
- Chamomile tea, with a little honey
- Mint tea, with a little honey
- Filtered or sparkling water with a little bit of apple cider vinegar added

Stage 2

Continue eating as in stage 1, and add:

- Raw egg yolks (see sidebar), then soft-cooked eggs
- Stews that meet all other criteria for stage 2
- Gravlax (cured fish)
- Homemade yogurt or sour cream
- Fresh herbs
- Clarified butter
- Coconut oil
- Honey-ginger drops (to stabilize blood sugar)

Fiber

Fiber may irritate a weak intestinal wall and can, for some Gapsters, create an obstruction in the intestine that is the perfect dwelling for undesirable microbes. For these reasons, the first stages of the intro diet are very low in fiber. You can eat low-fiber vegetables, but they must be cooked until quite tender. As you progress through the stages, you will gradually be able to eat more types of vegetables, and to eat them raw.

At some point during your progression through the full GAPS diet, you will probably be able to eat certain legumes, such as lentils and white beans, but they must first be soaked and cooked according to the directions in this book (see pages 72 and 73). Not until you have gotten rid of the worst of your GAPS symptoms will you be able to start getting all of the fiber that is generally recommended.

Ask your GAPS practitioner (see page 48) for advice on your fiber intake as you progress through the stages of the diet.

Stage 3

Continue eating as in stage 2, and add:

- Scrambled eggs
- Pancakes
- Homemade kefir in small amounts (start with 1 tsp/5 mL and increase gradually)
- Asparagus
- Cabbage
- Celery
- Celery root (celeriac)
- Sauerkraut
- Avocados
- Increasing amounts of animal fats

Stage 4

Continue eating as in stage 3, and add:

- Braised and grilled meat and fish
- Cold-pressed olive oil, unheated
- Freshly pressed vegetable juice (see page 204)
- Nuts and seeds (except Brazil nuts and pistachios), soaked and dried as directed on page 74
- Bread and crackers baked from nuts, seeds and kernels

Stage 5

Continue eating as in stage 4, and add:

- Fresh lettuce and peeled cucumbers
- All other raw vegetables
- Applesauce
- Freshly pressed fruit juice added to fresh vegetable juice (a maximum of 50% fruit juice), but wait on lemon juice
- Spices

Stage 6

Continue eating as in stage 5, and add:

- Peeled apples with a little honey
- Baked goods (cakes, pies, cookies) made with honey or dried fruit as a sweetener
- Brazil nuts and pistachios
- Capers

> ### Did You Know?
> **Eat Plenty of Fat**
> While on the GAPS diet, including the intro diet from stage 2, be sure to consume plenty of saturated fat, such as clarified butter and coconut oil (as of stage 2) and increasing amounts of animal fats (as of stage 3), as well as cold-pressed olive oil (as of stage 4) and a good fish oil supplement (following your practitioner's guidance). For more information on fat, see "The Skinny on Fat," page 36.

> ### Did You Know?
> **Drink Stock or Bone Broth Every Day**
> When on the intro diet, drink stock several times a day and add a poached egg or egg yolk to it when you can (once you are in stage 2). When you progress to the full GAPS diet, replace the stock with bone broth, which has a more potent medicinal effect.

Recipes for the Intro Diet

Stage 1	Baked Pumpkin or Squash (page 77) Beef Vegetable Soup (page 110) Cauliflower Chicken Stock (page 106) Chamomile Tea (page 205) Chicken or Veal Stock (page 102) Fish Stock (page 103) Fish Stock with Shrimp (page 105) Ginger Tea (page 205) Kefir whey (page 94) if you started with the full diet and have been using kefir whey for a while Mediterranean Stock (page 107) Sauerkraut brine (pages 84 and 86) Vallentino's Favorite Drink (page 206) Yogurt whey (page 92)
Stage 2	Clarified Butter (page 68) Fish Soup with Fennel (page 108) Ginger Drops (page 257) Gravlax (page 121) Hearty Chicken Stew (page 142) Lamb and Cabbage Stew (page 145) Mashed Root Vegetables (page 181) Meatball Stew with Spinach and Celery Root (page 146) Mushroom Fish Sauce (page 183) Stock with Poached Egg (page 104) Turkey, Mushroom and Spinach Stew (page 143) Veal Stew (page 144) Yogurt or Sour Cream (page 92)
Stage 3	Beef or Veal Liver Pâté (variation, page 126) Cauliflower Soup (variation, page 111) Chicken Liver Pâté (page 125) Corned Tongue in Mushroom Sauce (page 162) Creamed Celery Root (page 175) Duck or Goose Fat (page 70) Kefir (page 94) in small amounts Lumpfish Roe with Avocado (page 122) Lunch Wraps with Salmon Filling for Stage 3 or Chicken Filling for Stage 3 (variations, page 115) Sauerkraut (pages 84 and 86) Sour Cream Pancakes (page 217) Spinach Pancakes (page 118) Tomato Soup (variation, page 113) White Asparagus with Lemon Butter (variation, page 171) Zucchini Pancakes (page 119)
Stage 4	Aïoli (variation, page 188) Almond and Seed Crackers (page 200) Almond Cream (page 230) Baked Salmon (variation, page 149) Beet Chips (page 198) Bolognese Sauce (page 158)

Stage 4 (continued)	Carrot and Zucchini Spaghetti (page 182) Carrot Juice (page 206) Fish Cakes (variation, page 151) Fried Herring (page 148) GAPS-Friendly Pizza with a Crispy Crust (page 160; see tip) GAPS Smoothie (page 209) Green Juice (page 207) Guacamole (variation, page 139) Italian Salad (page 133) Mayonnaise (page 187) Meatballs (page 157) Nut and Seed Bread (page 270) Nuts and Seeds (page 74) Oil and Vinegar Dressing (page 192) Oven-Baked Vegetables (variation, page 180) Ravigote Sauce (page 189) Rémoulade (page 189) Root Vegetable Patties (page 136) Salted Almonds (page 201) Sesame Crisps (page 199) Slow-Braised Pork Hocks (page 156) Veal Heart Casserole (page 166)
Stage 5	Apple Pork (page 154) Applesauce (page 219) Carrot, Apple and Celery Juice (page 208) GAPS Sushi (page 123) Horseradish Cream (page 184) Lunch Wraps with Salmon Filling (page 114) Marinated Sun-Dried Tomatoes (page 197) Sweet-and-Sour Red Cabbage (page 172) Veal Tails in Red Wine (page 165) Vitello Tornado (page 130)
Stage 6	Almond Tuiles (page 252) Baked Salmon (page 149) Banana Bread (page 271) Banana Pancakes (page 216) Berry Iced Kefir (page 232) Brussels Sprout and Apple Salad (page 135) Carrot and Avocado Smoothie (page 210) Cauliflower Couscous (page 174) Flavored Honey (page 78) Fried Liver with Onions and Mushrooms (page 159) Kefir Eggnog (page 211) Lamb Liver Pâté (page 128) Lemon Buttercream (page 262) Lemon Tea (page 205) Peanut Butter Sauce (page 185) Quick Strawberry Ice Cream (page 232) Sweet-and-Sour Pork (page 155) Tarte Tatin à la GAPS (page 238) White Asparagus with Lemon Butter (page 171)

Die-Off

Whether you start with the intro diet or the full diet, you may experience "die-off." This phenomenon, also known as a healing crisis or the Herxheimer reaction, occurs in the course of many different diets and in other forms of treatment, too. What "dies off" are harmful intestinal microbes, because they are no longer being fed by sugar and starch and because they are being overpowered by probiotics — that is, the beneficial bacteria. When harmful microbes and other toxic substances die faster than your body can manage to get rid of them, old symptoms may flare up or you may experience completely new ones. Old traumas of a physical and/or mental nature may reemerge.

Examples of physical symptoms that can occur as a result of die-off include headaches, fatigue, difficulty concentrating, dizziness, nightmares, sleeplessness, eczema, hives, acne, muscle or tendon pain, toothaches and unusual amounts

Facebook, GAPS Diet Group, March 2, 2016

Jill
Can anyone tell me whether the intro diet has helped them and whether it has resulted in a noticeable change in any way?

Dina
No more candida!

Paige
Yes. I had a terrible and painful rash on my face. It might have gone away under any circumstances while I was on the full GAPS diet, but there is no doubt in my mind that I needed the intense healing of the intro diet. It took 3 months in stage 2, after which I flew through the remaining stages. I am currently still on the full diet.

Elizabeth
I think it helped me to clearly establish which food products were giving me problems (whereas on the full diet I would probably just have consumed those products).

Kelly
Yup! It helped all of us. The only thing I regret is how fast we flew through it. We managed really well when following the intro, but then around stage 5 we started increasing the pace and got lost. So be careful! When you get to where you start frying and baking, etc., you risk forgetting the soups, which really just amounts to being on a paleo diet. We're going to try giving it a go again next summer.

of dental tartar, as well as scars that flare up and become wounds, to later disappear without a trace.

Experiencing die-off is actually a good sign, but it shouldn't be too severe! You are detoxifying and will most likely feel much better once you have gotten through it.

Although I personally did not experience severe die-off as I detoxified, some people have related very unpleasant die-off symptoms. It all depends on the amount of toxins in your body and how intense your consumption of probiotics is. The box on page 28 explains the best way to escalate your intake of beneficial bacteria.

It may be a good idea to plan on starting the diet during a period when you can allow yourself to feel a little under the weather without having to manage your normal day-to-day routines — a time when you can relax, get a lot of sleep, take baths, go for walks and so on. In other words, choose a time when you can take a few days to focus on yourself and your detoxification process.

Experiencing die-off is actually a good sign, but it shouldn't be too severe! You are detoxifying and will most likely feel much better once you have gotten through it.

The Full GAPS Diet

When you're on the full diet, you can, in theory, eat anything from the food lists on pages 30–32. In the beginning, avoid foods that you know you cannot tolerate; after a while, as the diet progresses, you can try testing them out with small portions at a time to see whether you have become able to tolerate them.

Although the progression and duration of the full GAPS diet will be different for everyone, below you'll find some basic guidelines on the foods you should be sure to include as you work your way through it.

Fermented Foods

Eat fermented foods every day, as they provide beneficial bacteria. To avoid feeling too sick as a result of die-off (see page 26), start with very small portions and increase your intake gradually, as explained in the box on page 28. Recipes for fermented foods can be found on pages 84–95.

Bone Broth

Consume bone broth every day while you are on the full diet, to help heal your intestinal wall. Try to drink it with each meal, and add it to your hot dishes. Broth made solely of beef bones is hard to get down in terms of taste, but it is wonderful as a base in a soup or casserole, or in minced meat. For a broth more suitable for drinking, try a mixture of beef, veal,

Did You Know?

Drinking Bone Broth or Stock Is a Must

If you are not drinking bone broth (or stock while on the intro diet) several times a day, every day, then you are not on the GAPS diet! If you have problems tolerating it, I cannot stress enough the importance of tending to the problem and getting help from a GAPS practitioner (see page 48).

How to Increase Your Intake of Probiotics

Start with 1 to 2 teaspoons (5 to 10 mL) of sauerkraut brine (see recipe, page 85) per day; don't make the mistake of being overconfident and eating more than that. Probiotics can have a very strong effect, and you want to make sure to curb any unpleasant symptoms. After a few days without any die-off symptoms, you can continue adding 1 teaspoon (5 mL) at a time until you are consuming 1 to 1$\frac{2}{3}$ cups (250 to 400 mL) of brine a day. Sip the brine as a refreshing drink or add it to soup.

Whey from homemade yogurt (page 92) can supplement the sauerkraut brine; as with brine, add it into your diet gradually, starting with 1 teaspoon (5 mL) or following the recommendations of your GAPS practitioner. Wait to use kefir whey (page 94) until you have been on the diet for a while, as it is a potent probiotic. Both types of whey make a great addition to stocks, bone broths, soups, fresh juices and smoothies.

Do not add probiotics to food, such as soup, that is above 109°F (43°C) or the beneficial bacteria will die. (The same thing applies if you are opening up a probiotics supplement and adding the powder to food.)

chicken, duck, pork, lamb and/or game bones (and for fish bone broth, try a mix of fish bones). Bone broth for the GAPS diet should be slow-cooked for 12 to 72 hours (except for fish bone broth, which should cook for 4 to 24 hours).

Animal Foods

Animal foods have a crucial function in the body: they supply our cells with the nutrients needed to maintain the body's structure: the skeleton, connective tissue, cartilage, muscles, nerves, skin, and so on. These nutrients are especially high in bone broth cooked from bones, cartilage, connective tissue and marrow.

Unlike many diets, the GAPS diet does not focus on high-priced lean cuts of meat. Instead, it recommends that you prioritize eating organ meats, such as heart, kidney and liver, which are extremely high in many important micro-nutrients. Liver, for example, contains much more absorbable vitamin B_{12} and iron than any other food. (If you don't like liver, sneak it into minced meat to disguise its flavor while reaping its benefits.) You can eat other cuts of meat as well, but choose meat with the natural fat still on it and eat the fat! Purchase poultry and fish with the skin on, and eat the skin, too.

Vegetables

In addition to lots of high-fat meat, the GAPS diet encourages us to eat lots of vegetables. Well-prepared vegetables give your meals an array of wonderful flavor nuances, fill you up and

Did You Know?

Save Your Scraps!
If you don't have enough appetite to eat everything on your plate, put the scraps in the freezer together with the bones for the next batch of bone broth and throw your leftovers in the soup you make with the broth!

contribute slow-burning carbohydrates as well as vitamins, minerals and other micronutrients.

Fresh herbs, such as parsley, chives, basil and dill, are another wonderful way to add flavor and micronutrients to your meals, whether cooked into the meal itself or sprinkled on top. The recipes in this book call for plenty of fresh herbs, which can usually be found in the produce section of the grocery store even during the winter months.

Freshly Pressed Juices

You can get a lot of nutrients from raw vegetables by juicing them, and juicing removes the fiber, which is difficult for many Gapsters to digest (see "Fiber," page 22). Moreover, freshly pressed vegetable juices help the body with detoxification. Fruit can be added to your juice for flavor and sweetness, but fruit juice should make up no more than 50% of the total because of its sugar content.

Note that store-bought vegetable juices cannot be used as a detoxifier, as they have been sterilized with either heat or high-pressure pasteurization, both of which kill microorganisms so efficiently that the beneficial nutrients are also destroyed. Moreover, store-bought juices can contain a lot of "mystery" ingredients that you don't want to put into your body.

Many retail outlets, mall kiosks and even gyms now offer fresh vegetable juices, juiced right in front of you while you wait. But if you're going to be drinking fresh juices regularly, a juicer would be a good investment, so you can prepare your own juices at home. Recipes for juice are on pages 206–208.

Recipes for juice are on pages 206–208.

Did You Know?

Sweeteners

Use ripe fresh and dried fruit as sweeteners while on the GAPS diet. As a monosaccharide, honey is also acceptable in moderate amounts; raw honey even contains antimicrobial properties (as long as it remains unheated). You may use a little fresh stevia (not the processed kind), but do not use syrups, exotic sugars or artificial sweeteners.

Complementary Benefits

In her article "One Man's Meat Is Another Man's Poison," Natasha Campbell-McBride explains the fundamental difference between animal foods and plant foods as far as their effects on health. In brief, the article's message is that there are two types of food:

1. Animal foods, which renew the body's cells so they can build and maintain its structure.
2. Vegetables, which work as cleansers.

The article also explains why there is no use in putting everyone on an identical diet: everyone's needs are different, and one's needs can vary on an individual level at different times of life. The needs of someone who is healthy and symptom-free, for example, are very different from those of someone who is ill.

What to Eat on the Full GAPS Diet

A	Almonds Anchovies Animal fat (beef, chicken, duck, goose, lamb, pork, etc.) Apple juice (not from concentrate) Apples	Apricots Artichokes Asparagus Avocado oil, cold-pressed Avocados
B	Bacon (with no additives other than salt) Bananas, ripe Beans, pole (such as green, yellow and scarlet) Beef[1] Beef fat Beets	Bell peppers Berries (all kinds) Bok choy Brazil nuts Broccoli (introduce stalks gradually) Brussels sprouts Butter (clarified or whole)
C	Cabbage Cacao (raw chocolate; introduce gradually) Capers Carrots Cashews Cauliflower (introduce stalks gradually) Caviar (without color) Celery Celery root (celeriac) Cheese, ripe and aged[2] Cherries Chia seeds (introduce gradually) Chicken[1] Chicken fat Chile peppers Chives Cider	Clarified butter Clementines Cocoa butter Cocoa powder, unsweetened (introduce gradually) Coconut, fresh and dried[3] Coconut milk, preferably homemade Coconut oil, cold-pressed Coconut water Cod roe, fresh Coffee, weak, from real beans (introduce gradually) Cottage cheese, homemade Crab Crayfish Cucumbers
D	Dates (without additives) Duck[1] Duck fat	
E	Eggplant Eggs Escargot (snails)	
F	Fennel Fermented vegetables Figs Fish, fresh, frozen or canned in oil or water, except tuna	Flax seeds Foie gras Frog's legs
G	Garlic Ghee, homemade Ginger Goat[1]	Goose[1] Goose fat Grapefruit Grapes
H	Hazelnuts Hemp seeds (introduce gradually) Herbal teas[4]	Herbs (all kinds, fresh and dried) Honey
J	Juice[5]	

K	Kale Kefir, fermented for 24 hours Kimchi Kiwifruit	Kohlrabi (introduce gradually) Kombucha (fermented tea), also known as kvass Kumquats
L	Lamb[1] Lamb fat Leafy green vegetables (all kinds) Leeks Lemons Lentils (introduce gradually)	Lettuce (all kinds) Licorice root Lima beans (introduce gradually) Limes Lumpfish roe
M	Macadamia nuts Mangos Mead made from honey Melons Mushrooms	Mussels Mustard, Dijon (with only GAPS-approved additives) Mutton[1]
N	Napa cabbage Nectarines	Nut or seed butter (such as almond butter, cashew butter or tahini)

O	Olive oil, cold-pressed
	Olives (without sugar or other unsuitable
	   ingredients)
	Onions
	Oranges
		Organ meat (heart, kidney, liver,
		   sweetbreads, tongue)[1]
		Ox[1]
		Oysters

P	Palm oil, cold-pressed Papayas Parsley root (introduce gradually) Passion fruit Peaches Peanut butter (without additives) Peanut oil, cold-pressed Peanuts Pears Peas, green Pecans	Peppers, bell and chile Pheasant[1] Pine nuts Pineapple Plums Pork[1] Pork fat Pork lard Prunes (without sugar or other additives) Pumpkin Pumpkin seeds
Q	Quail[1]	Quince
R	Radishes Raisins	Rapeseed oil, cold-pressed Rhubarb

S	Sauerkraut, homemade
	Sausages (with no additives other than
	   herbs and spices)
	Seaweed (introduce gradually), except
	   algae and carrageenan
	Sesame oil, cold-pressed
	Sesame seeds
	Shellfish
	Shrimp
		Sour cream, fermented for 24 hours
		Sparkling water
		Spices (all kinds, whole and ground,
		   without additives)
		Spinach
		Split peas (introduce gradually)
		Squash, winter and summer
		Stevia (only fresh and in limited
		   amounts)
		Sunflower seeds

T	Tangerines Tea,[5] weak (introduce gradually) Tomato juice (with no additives except salt) Tomato purée (with no additives except salt) Tomato salsa, homemade	Tomatoes Tomatoes, crushed (in glass jars) Turkey[1] Turkey fat Turnips (once healing has taken place)[6]

U	Ugli fruit	
V	Vanilla beans or pure vanilla extract[7] Veal[1] Venison and other game[1]	Vinegar (all kinds, so long as there is no added sugar) Vodka (on rare occasions)
W	Walnuts Watercress Whisky (on rare occasions)	White beans (introduce gradually), except cannellini Wine, dry
Y	Yellow summer squash	Yogurt, fermented for 24 hours
Z	Zucchini	

1 Eat all meat with its natural fat, and poultry with its skin.

2 Eat only hard cheese, blue cheese, red culture cheese and white cheese (from cows, sheep or goats). The cheese must have aged for at least 30 days and should contain no additives other than a bacterial culture.

3 For shredded coconut, grate a fresh coconut or buy unsweetened coarsely shredded coconut of good quality. It is possible to purchase some inexpensive but very poor-quality shredded coconut; that won't do.

4 Teabags often contain various substances that are not allowed on the GAPS diet. Use pure tea leaves and only use teabags when you know what their exact contents are.

5 Juice should be freshly squeezed from vegetables and allowed ripe fruit; homemade or store-bought pure juice with no added sugar, not from concentrate, is also acceptable.

6 The extent to which turnips can be tolerated is very individual. Give them a try once you are well into the GAPS diet.

7 Vanilla extract may contain additives that are not suitable for the GAPS diet; if you do use it, make sure to use only pure vanilla extract, and read the label to make sure it contains only vanilla, water and alcohol, with no other additives.

Wait Before Eating Certain Foods

Some foods and beverages can be hard for weak stomachs to handle, so wait to try these until you are well into the diet:

- Beans, white and lima
- Cacao (raw chocolate)
- Cauliflower and broccoli stalks
- Chia seeds
- Cocoa, unsweetened
- Coffee
- Hemp seeds
- Kohlrabi
- Lentils
- Parsley root
- Seaweed
- Split peas
- Tea, black
- Turnips

Did You Know?

Can I Eat This?

Are you in doubt as to whether a prepared food product is GAPS-friendly? Check the ingredient list. If it contains sugar, starch, partly hydrogenated plant oil or additives with terms you are not familiar with, then skip that product. For meats, find a butcher you can trust and who says their products are made without starch, sugar or additives.

What to Avoid on the GAPS Diet

The key omissions in the GAPS diet, to avoid feeding harmful bacteria in the gut, are sugar (and other sweeteners, such as maple syrup and agave nectar) and starch (found in grains and some vegetables). In addition, processed foods should generally be avoided. They do not contain nutrients like real food does. Furthermore, heavy-handed processing often diminishes the taste, consistency and appearance of the food products, and these deficits are then concealed with all sorts of GAPS-unfriendly additives.

What to Avoid on the GAPS Diet		
A	Adzuki beans Agar-agar Agave nectar Algae	Amaranth Arrowroot (used as a starch) Aspartame Astragalus tea
B	Baking powder and any kind of 　raising agent Baking soda Barley Barley malt syrup Bean flour Bean sprouts Beer Black-eyed peas	Broth or bouillon (store-bought: liquid, 　cubes or granulated) Brown rice syrup Brown sugar Buckwheat Bulgur Butter, spreadable Butter substitutes Buttermilk
C	Candy with sugar and additives Canned vegetables Cannellini beans Canola oil Carob Carrageenan Cereals, ready-to-eat Cheese, fresh and unaged 　(such as feta or mozzarella) Cheese spread Chestnut flour Chestnuts Chewing gum Chickpeas (garbanzo beans) Chicory root Chips[1]	Chocolate Cocoa powder, sweetened Coffee, instant Confectioners' sugar Cookies, store-bought Corn Corn flour Corn syrup Cornstarch Cottage cheese, store-bought Couscous Crackers, store-bought Cream Cream cheese Crispbread
D	Dairy products, processed[2] Date syrup	Demerara sugar Dextrose
F	Fava beans Fermented dairy products, store-bought Fish, canned, packed in sauce	FOS (fructooligosaccharides) Fructose extracted from corn Fruit, canned
G	Granulated sugar	
I	Ice cream, store-bought	Icing sugar

J	Jaggery Jam/jelly Jerusalem artichokes	Juice made from concentrate Juice with added sugar
K	Ketchup, store-bought	
L	Liqueur	Lucuma powder
M	Maca root Madeira Maple syrup Margarine Marmalade Mead made from sugar	Meat products with additives Milk (cow's, goat's, sheep's) Millet Molasses Mung beans
N	Noodles NutraSweet (aspartame)	Nuts, store-bought, salted and/or roasted
O	Oat milk Oats	Okra
P	Palm sugar Parsnips Pasta Pea flour Pearl sugar Pectin (as an additive) Plantains	Plant oils that are not cold-pressed Port Potatoes Powdered sugar Preserved fruits Psyllium husk
Q	Quinoa	
R	Rapadura Red beans Rice Rice crackers	Rice milk Root vegetable chips with additives Rye
S	Saccharin Sauces, ready-made Sausage with additives Seeds, store-bought, salted and/or roasted Semolina Sherry Soft drinks Sour cream, commercially processed Soybeans	Soy milk Soy sauce Spelt Starfruit[3] Stevia (except for fresh stevia, in limited amounts) Sukrin Sweet potatoes Sweeteners[4]
T	Tapioca Tea, instant Tofu	Triticale Tuna[5]
V	Vanilla sugar or vanilla powder Vegetable oils that are not cold-pressed and any oil labeled "cooking oil"	Vinegar with added sugar
W	Wheat and all components (germ, bran) Whey, store-bought, liquid or powder	White sugar
X	Xylitol	

| Y | | Yacón syrup | | Yeast |
| | | Yams | | Yogurt, store-bought |

1 *"Chips" refers to all forms of commercially manufactured snacks, including salted and salty-sweet snacks such as potato chips, corn chips, pretzels, cheese doodles and much more. Even organic root vegetable chips may be produced with additives and/or may contain potatoes.*

2 *There are many processed dairy products that are not suitable for individuals on the GAPS diet, including fresh cheese, feta cheese and store-bought cottage cheese. Milk kefir can be purchased for the sake of taste and consistency, but because it has been either heated or exposed to high-pressure treatment before reaching the shelves, it is not suitable to use as a probiotic supplement (as can be done when it is homemade).*

3 *Starfruit (also known as carambola) should not be consumed if you have kidney disease. Worldwide, there have been several reports of sudden deaths occurring among kidney patients after they have consumed starfruit, which contains substances that they absolutely cannot tolerate.*

4 *All sweeteners (except for dried fruit, honey and fresh stevia) should be avoided on the GAPS diet. This list contains only a selection of common sweeteners. There are as many as 100 natural and processed sweeteners, and over 50 sweetener brands.*

5 *Tuna should generally be avoided due to its high content of heavy metal.*

The Transition Diet

The GAPS diet is usually followed for at least 2 years, and you must have been symptom-free for at least 6 months before you start phasing out of it. Start the transition slowly! Begin by adding new potatoes to your meals, and then sourdough bread. Gradually try other forms of starch. As long as no symptoms recur, you're good to go; if you experience a relapse of symptoms after eating a certain food, remove that food from your diet once more.

Do not assume that you can now simply start to devour food products like packaged macaroni and cheese, sugar-laden commercial baked goods or frozen TV dinners. You must always be sure to eat properly — that is to say, real food made from quality ingredients. On the other hand, at this point, you can probably go berserk every now and then without actually getting sick. Experiment a little and make note of your experiences.

If you experience a relapse of symptoms after eating a certain food, remove that food from your diet once more.

Facebook, GAPS Diet Group, November 7, 2015

Joiel

I just want to share our good news with all of you. We've managed to reach the other side! We have followed the GAPS diet meticulously, including the intro diet, for a total of 5 years while slowly incorporating non-GAPS food into our diet during the last 2 years. And now my son's PDD-NOS diagnosis (belongs to the category of autism spectrum disorders) is officially gone, he no longer has any symptoms or special needs that need to be taken into consideration, and he can eat ordinary American food without any problems. I have been very thankful for this development for a long time! And this summer I am grateful for having to do less cooking and cleaning of dishes. *It can be done. Recovery is possible.*

The Skinny on Fat

Fat contributes to flavor, it binds food together and it fills you up, providing a natural curb on how much it is physically possible for you to eat. But what types of fat are best when you want to take care of your health?

All forms of fat contain three types of fatty acids: saturated, monounsaturated and polyunsaturated. If a fatty substance contains mostly saturated fatty acids, we simply call it a saturated fat even though it also contains the other types of fatty acids. Olive oil contains mostly monounsaturated fatty acids, so we call it a monounsaturated oil. And so on.

Because of their chemical structure, *saturated fats*, such as coconut oil, butter and veal fat, are solid at room temperature and when refrigerated, melting only when heated. They can tolerate exposure to oxygen, high temperatures and light without any risk of their chemical structure changing and becoming harmful to your health.

In contrast, *polyunsaturated fats*, such as corn oil, sunflower oil and grapeseed oil, are fluid in the refrigerator and at room temperature. Their chemical structure is much "looser" than that of saturated fats; therefore, it can easily change, which it does when it is exposed to light, oxygen or high temperatures.

Monounsaturated fats, such as duck fat and olive oil, fall in between saturated and polyunsaturated fats. They are semifluid at room temperature but can become solid when exposed to cold. They tolerate exposure to heat, light and oxygen without becoming harmful; however, olive oil's helpful, health-promoting compounds are destroyed by heat.

> *The type of fat you choose is a key component of the healing process when you are following the GAPS diet.*

Choosing Fats for the GAPS Diet

Because the type of fat you choose is a key component of the healing process when you are following the GAPS diet, I will now briefly sum up what types of fats are good for cold food and what types are good for making hot food.

Fats for Cold Food

While all fats *can* be used for cold foods, some *must* be used for cold foods. In general, eat plant oils cold (except for coconut oil). Use them in salad dressings, cold sauces, mayonnaise and dips. Some monounsaturated plant oils can be used in a pinch to prepare hot food (see below), but do not cook with plant oils that are mainly polyunsaturated.

When polyunsaturated fatty acids are exposed to high temperatures, their chemical structure is altered, and they become damaging to your health. The more polyunsaturated fatty acids a fat contains, the more vulnerable it is to high temperatures and the less suitable it is for heating. Thus, there are no polyunsaturated fats that are suitable for preparing hot food.

There are no polyunsaturated fats that are suitable for preparing hot food.

Fats for Hot Food

Fats that can be used to prepare hot food are:

- all animal fats, whether saturated or monounsaturated;
- butter, clarified butter and ghee (Indian clarified fermented butter);
- cold-pressed coconut oil, palm oil and palm seed oil (plant oils that are mainly saturated fat).

Saturated Fats

Saturated fatty acids do not change their chemical structure when heated and retain their ability to heal the body and mind. To maintain good health, it is therefore best to choose this type of fat for cooking. (See "Why Saturated Fat?" on page 39 for further discussion of this somewhat controversial topic.)

Monounsaturated Fats

The suitability of monounsaturated fats for heating depends on what proportion of polyunsaturated fatty acids they contain in relation to their monounsaturated and saturated fatty acid content. All monounsaturated animal fats are suitable for heating because their proportion of polyunsaturated fatty acids is low. But what about monounsaturated plant oils? While all of these oils can be used to prepare hot food *if necessary* (when you really have no other options, such as animal fat), it is important to choose an oil with the lowest possible polyunsaturated fat content. The lower the amount of polyunsaturated fatty acid, the less harmful the oil is when heated.

Did You Know?

Olive Oil

If you must use a monounsaturated plant oil for cooking, olive oil is the best choice. Keep in mind, however, that olive oil contains many beneficial substances that disappear when it is heated; to reap the full benefit of these nutrients, consume olive oil cold.

Composition and Use of Various Fats

	COMPOSITION			USE	
	Mainly saturated	Mainly mono-unsaturated	Mainly poly-unsaturated	For hot food	For cold food
ANIMAL FATS					
Butter	•			•	•
Beef fat	•			•	•
Chicken fat		•		•	•
Duck fat		•		•	•
Goose fat		•		•	•
Lamb fat	•			•	•
Pork fat (drippings)	•	•		•	•
Pork lard (solid)		•		•	•
Veal fat	•			•	•
PLANT OILS*					
Almond oil		•			•
Avocado oil		•			•
Cashew nut oil			•		•
Coconut oil	•			•	•
Corn oil			•		•
Cottonseed oil			•		•
Flaxseed oil			•		•
Grapeseed oil			•		•
Hempseed oil			•		•
Macadamia oil		•		•	•
Olive oil		•		•	•
Palm oil	•			•	•
Palm seed oil	•			•	•
Peanut oil		•		•	•
Pecan oil		•			•
Pumpkin seed oil			•		•
Rapeseed oil		•		•	•
Safflower oil			•		•
Sesame oil		•	•	•	•
Soy oil			•		•
Sunflower oil			•		•
Thistle oil			•		•
Walnut oil			•		•
Wheat germ oil			•		•

* All plant oils must be cold-pressed; otherwise, they are already ruined at the time of purchase.

In Summary

- Use animal fat, including butter, and cold-pressed coconut oil or palm oil for hot food and for baking.

- Use monounsaturated plant oils for cold sauces and dressings. Use them in hot dishes only if you have no other options on hand, in which case olive oil is the best choice.

- Use polyunsaturated plant oils in small amounts as flavorings in cold sauces, dips and dressings. These oils should be kept in dark-colored, airtight bottles in the refrigerator.

- Use fat from animals that have grazed, and use plant oils that have been cold-pressed. Avoid using cheap food oils altogether.

Fish Oil

Fish oil is unsuitable for cooking because of its strong fishy flavor, among other factors. But we still need it in our diet! For that reason, fish oil, which contains polyunsaturated omega-3 fatty acids, is one of the few dietary supplements recommended in the GAPS diet on a regular basis. Find a good-quality brand.

When you are cooking fish, the oil in the meat can tolerate being heated without adverse effects — it isn't nearly as vulnerable as oil that has been extracted from the fish. So you can simmer, fry or bake fatty fish without concern. One delicious way to get fish oil is to eat salmon in the form of gravlax; see the recipe on page 121.

Why Saturated Fat?

Humans have thrived on animal fat, both saturated and monounsaturated, for millennia. The human body is made up of 70% water; the remaining 30% is half protein and half fat. Our bodies' cells need constant upkeep and repair, and that maintenance requires building materials in the form of the protein and fat provided by animal food. Saturated and monounsaturated fats contribute to creating and maintaining cells throughout the body — in the brain, the muscles, the immune system and so on. A good part of every cell in the body is composed of fat.

Fat also helps us absorb protein and prevents toxic nitrogen buildup, which can be the result of eating too much lean red meat. Saturated fat is an important component of our nerve fibers and a number of our organs. If you are interested in learning more about saturated fat and its contributions to optimal health, several excellent resources on the subject are listed in the References on page 276.

When we analyze human fat cells, it becomes clear that saturated fat is the type that most resembles them and is therefore the most suitable for maintaining them. So it is important to regularly consume saturated fat, from meat, butter and coconut oil. Don't make do with lean meat, and don't trim off the fat; to help your body heal and rebuild, eat meat *with* its natural fat.

Debunking the Anti–Saturated Fat Campaign

Perhaps you are about to choke on your skim milk. Saturated fat? It has been frowned upon by the experts since the 1950s!

That's true: for more than six decades, researchers, doctors and nutritional advisers have been telling us that eating fat makes you fat, and that dietary fat is the root of many diseases. This belief has become the foundation for many discussions on food and has permeated all types of media, from professional journals to weekly newspapers, and every recommendation by professional practitioners, be they established or alternative. The consistent message has been that saturated fat promotes cardiovascular disease, increases your cholesterol numbers and causes weight gain.

Throughout the years, a tiny number of specialists have voiced their opposition to this "truth," and in recent years more and more experts have begun to get on board with refuting the premise that saturated fat is detrimental to our health.

New York author Nina Teicholz is an investigative journalist who wrote the 2014 book *The Big Fat Surprise: Why Butter, Meat & Cheese Belong in a Healthy Diet.* The book explains how we have gotten to the point where we believe that saturated fat is damaging to our health, despite the fact that humans subsisted largely on it for centuries without contracting the lifestyle diseases we are so familiar with today. In an attempt to determine what has been behind the political and financial trends regarding fat since the 1950s, Teicholz spent 9 years poring through research papers, reading them in their entirety and noting when the conclusion reached by the study authors seemed to state the exact opposite of what their data indicated.

Teicholz's book, along with science journalist Gary Taubes's bulky 2007 book *Good Calories, Bad Calories: Fats, Carbs and the Controversial Science of Diet and Health*, confirms what researchers like Mary Enig of the United States and Uffe Ravnskov of Denmark have claimed for years. As Ravnskov writes in his 2010 book *Hvorfor et højt kolesteroltal er nyttigt* (*Why Having a High Cholesterol Number Is Advantageous*): "Convincing half the world that saturated fat is damaging to your health is nothing less than a masterpiece of deception." Enig and Ravnskov warn of a dire outcome for human health if we continue to follow the current official dietary guidelines.

In her 2007 book, *Put Your Heart in Your Mouth*, which explains how heart disease arises, Natasha Campbell-McBride writes that, in her opinion, we need natural fats from natural foods and that saturated and monounsaturated fats should comprise most of our fat intake. The simplified notion that fat is fattening is completely wrong. It is processed carbohydrates that make us fat, she says.

Did You Know?

The True Culprits
Specialists who study fat have declared that the main culprits in the ongoing obesity and diabetes epidemics are sugar and refined grain products; "lite" products and processed food also contribute to wreaking havoc in the digestive system.

RESEARCH ROUNDUP

Fat Is Not the Enemy
Several other studies and books have recently emerged to dismantle the notion that saturated fats should be stamped as culprits. In 2008, a group of American researchers examined all the studies that dealt with low-fat diets and found no evidence that they improved health in any way. In 2013, a Swedish research group closely examined 16,000 low-fat studies and concluded that a lean diet was strategically inefficient in relation to diabetes and overweight. And in 2014, the Danish nutritional expert Arne Astrup established in a meta-analysis that there was no evidence that saturated fat increases the risk of cardiovascular disease.

Answers to Common Questions

Many people around the globe have found tremendous relief from their symptoms and illnesses after following the GAPS protocol for a while, but nothing is black and white, and that's certainly true when it comes to making major lifestyle changes. Sticking to a new diet can be hard work, both mentally and practically. However, the potential payoff may be very rewarding — or even life-changing.

It's only natural to have a ton of questions as you get started on the GAPS diet. Here, I've provided answers to some of the most common questions people have when diving in, to help you decide what is right for you in terms of turning all this information into action.

Q: How should I approach the GAPS diet if I have a food allergy or intolerance?

A: When your gut is depleted of various species of beneficial bacteria and, on top of that, you have an intestinal wall full of holes, you may develop food allergies and intolerances. Milk, eggs, gluten, nuts, shellfish, nightshade vegetables (such as tomatoes and peppers) and fruit are classic examples of foods that some people have an adverse reaction to, just as many people have an allergic reaction when exposed to pollen, animal dander or dust. Some food allergies and intolerances are due to genetic factors, but in many cases, allergic symptoms are caused by an unhealthy gut flora.

If you have such symptoms when you consume certain foods, avoid these products when you first begin to follow the diet. Focus on patching the holes in your intestinal wall, which happens the fastest when you follow the intro diet. As you progress further into the diet and start to heal, carefully try the foods again to see whether you have become able to tolerate them. Take your time doing so. Some reactions may surface several days or even weeks after you have consumed a specific food.

Lactose Intolerance

Like other sugars, lactose — the sugar naturally found in milk — consists of two carbohydrate molecules that are joined together. These must be split into two single molecules in

---

Milk, eggs, gluten, nuts, shellfish, nightshade vegetables (such as tomatoes and peppers) and fruit are classic examples of foods that some people have an adverse reaction to.

Did You Know?

Introduce Questionable Foods Cautiously

If you know you have a true allergy, don't even think about testing the food that provokes it. But if your allergic symptoms are not life-threatening and you suspect your reactions might stem from intestinal bacteria and a leaky gut, you can try questionable foods cautiously, with guidance and support from a GAPS practitioner you trust. To be on the safe side, test a little bit of the food on your skin (see "How to Test Your Sensitivity to Food Products," page 21) *before* ingesting it.

order to be digestible, and for that to happen, the enzyme lactase must be put into action. But lactase does not work alone; it is dependent on a specific collaborator: the beneficial bacteria known as physiological *E. coli*. If these bacteria do not reside in your gut, then lactase cannot split the lactose molecules, which means you cannot digest the sugar and it will remain in your intestine, where it may become food for harmful microbes, or it may find a leak in the gut wall through which it can escape. Once it slips into the bloodstream, where it does not belong, your immune system will react, causing a variety of unpleasant symptoms.

When you patch up your intestinal wall and simultaneously supplement your food with as many varied forms of beneficial bacteria as possible, many lactose-intolerant individuals can expect to be able to tolerate the following dairy products again: soured milk and cream (yogurt and sour cream that have been fermented for 24 hours), kefir, butter, aged cheeses and raw milk (see box, page 91). Later on, you may even be able to tolerate small amounts of fresh, high-quality full-fat milk and cream from grass-fed animals, but this is very individual.

You may be able to tolerate homemade yogurt very quickly, because you will be fermenting your yogurt for 24 hours — the amount of time it takes to become almost lactose-free. This is a lot longer than the fermentation period for store-bought yogurt. Once you can tolerate homemade yogurt, try homemade sour cream, then homemade kefir, followed by mature cheese (aged for at least 1 month).

Clarified butter is something you can eat from the very start of the diet because the milk substances have been strained off, leaving only butter oil. After a while, you will most likely be able to consume good-quality organic butter!

Gluten Intolerance

Many people who believe they are gluten-intolerant are actually unable to digest starch in general, thanks to GAPS. In other words, the problem may not be gluten, but rather the starch found in flours, grains, potatoes, pasta and other products. Consuming expensive gluten-free products produced from all sorts of creative forms of starch and sugar is seldom a constructive approach for Gapsters. So if you have tried a gluten-free diet and found no relief from your symptoms, try the GAPS diet instead!

If you belong to the small group of people who are truly allergic to gluten and therefore suffer from celiac disease, then unfortunately you cannot eat your way out of the allergy, but you may still feel better if you follow the GAPS diet.

Did You Know?

Probiotic Gold

The whey strained from homemade yogurt is pure probiotic gold that many people can use as a supplement to their diets from the very beginning. Use the sensitivity test on page 21 to see if you are ready to start consuming whey. If not, you can get your probiotics from sauerkraut brine and gradually from sauerkraut itself.

Real-World Testimonial

There are some things the diet cannot help you with, as such, but it can improve your health and make your body better able to handle different kinds of problems. I suffer from celiac disease, so the diet will improve my health but not restore it entirely.

— *Melissa B*

Q: Will I be able to cut back on my medications?

A: Many people who follow the GAPS diet find that they no longer need to take medication to subdue symptoms or prevent a decline in their physical or mental health. If you are hoping to reduce your dosage or stop taking medication altogether in tandem with your improvement while on the GAPS diet, do so only in consultation with your doctor! Every medication is different, as is its purpose, its effects and the degree to which it is vital. If you start feeling much better, you may be tempted to toss all your medication away, but don't do it! Summon up your patience and talk to your doctor about whether you might be able to gradually reduce your dosage, with an eye toward eventually ceasing the medication. Remember that healing takes time.

If you are hoping to reduce your dosage or stop taking medication altogether in tandem with your improvement while on the GAPS diet, do so only in consultation with your doctor.

Q: Should I take dietary supplements while on the GAPS diet?

A: Talk to your GAPS practitioner (see page 48) about any dietary supplements you might need. Don't go out and blindly purchase all sorts of expensive supplements until you know your specific needs. Many dietary supplements are ineffective when taken alone — they must work in collaboration with other substances in order to be absorbed by the body. Get advice from an expert in this area. For example, if your iron stores are low, you should look into the underlying cause rather than simply taking an iron supplement. Low iron stores are not always the result of low iron intake; in some cases, the body is unable to absorb iron because of a complicated GAPS-related issue. Some Gapsters suffer from unwanted intestinal bacteria that feed on iron — and feeding harmful microbes is not a good idea.

Don't go out and blindly purchase all sorts of expensive supplements until you know your specific needs.

Q: I am a picky eater. How can I possibly survive on the GAPS diet?

A: Perhaps you are reluctant to start the GAPS diet because you are finicky. It goes without saying that finicky people are seldom open to new taste experiences. They would rather go hungry for a while than eat something they don't want. So it's understandable if you are worried that the GAPS diet includes too many foods that you won't like and not enough foods that you do.

One thing it is very important to establish at the outset is that you might be a picky eater *because* you have GAPS.

Certain foods, such as vegetables, fruits, herbs, nuts and seeds, may literally leave a bad taste in your mouth. That's because harmful bacteria can exist in the mouth as well as in the intestine. When detoxifying substances, which these foods contain, meet toxic bacteria in the mouth, the detoxifiers start to attack the microbes, a reaction that can feel like stinging, scratching or burning in the mouth — which your brain may interpret as the food not tasting good.

If, on top of having this experience of a bad taste in your mouth, you are also dependent on sugar, then it's not surprising if you prefer sugar and other fast-burning carbohydrates to vegetables. Finicky people typically prefer foods such as bread, pasta, crackers, candy, chocolate and ice cream — all foods that contain starch or sugar, or both.

Picky Kids

There are various strategies you can use to get a finicky child to eat foods other than the ones they prefer, and if you have a picky child, you have probably heard them all. Whatever strategy you follow, it is important to ensure that everyone involved has a solid understanding that only GAPS-friendly food is to be served to your child, regardless of how they react. The longest I have heard of a child refusing to eat was a heartbreaking 9 days. But his parents didn't give up. Finally, the boy caved in and started shoveling in the food that was served.

Consider becoming a member of the Facebook group "GAPS Kids," where you can find plenty of invaluable support and advice.

When you understand the connection between an unhealthy gut flora and being finicky, it becomes clear that you are dealing with a vicious cycle: the foods you love are the ones that are feeding the harmful bacteria in your gut and mouth, and the proliferation of these microbes is causing the bad taste in your mouth when you try to eat healthier foods. Yet the foods you reject are precisely the foods your body needs to help you stop being finicky. Give the GAPS diet a try, and over time you will notice that you are developing a taste for more and more types of food that you previously disliked. Once your gut heals, you will no longer need to think of yourself as a picky eater!

Real-World Testimonial

Changing the diet of my daughter, who is just under 4, when she was diagnosed with leaky gut and various other allergies was not easy. It took 3 difficult weeks until her taste buds and urge for good food changed. Don't give up! After a month we were astonished at how her sense of taste had changed. I'm talking about a child who would have gladly lived off fruit and toast for the rest of her life. Now she likes getting bone broth for breakfast, and she even eats liver without complaining.

— *Lora O*

Q: Will the GAPS diet help me achieve my ideal weight?

A: There are myriad diets with one paramount purpose: weight loss. That is not the focus of the GAPS diet. But if you have a weight problem, you will likely reach a weight that is suitable for you over the course of the diet. There are numerous examples of Gapsters who have either lost or gained weight as a bonus result of their detoxification process and gaining control of their inner biochemical condition.

Whether you wish to gain or lose weight, try not to focus on that goal. Instead, concentrate on detoxifying, repairing your intestinal wall and rebuilding health-strengthening gut flora through the GAPS diet.

If you are underweight and are worried about losing even more weight at the start of the diet — which is not uncommon — ask a GAPS practitioner (see page 48) for advice.

Q: Will the GAPS diet strengthen my immune system?

A: About 85% of the body's immune system is located inside the intestinal wall. So one of the joyous results of sealing up the leaks and healing your gut is seeing your immune function improve in response. You may well find that you are more resistant to colds and other viruses, fighting them off even as they lay low the people around you!

Q: What other lifestyle changes can I make to help heal my gut while I'm on the GAPS diet?

A: Natasha Campbell-McBride's book *Gut and Psychology Syndrome* describes additional proactive steps to consider while you're following the GAPS diet: getting enough sunlight (not under a scorching midday sun, of course); avoiding perfumes and additives in personal-care products; avoiding chemical substances in cleaning products and detergents; helping the detoxification process by taking enemas and detox baths; having a pet; and, in general, occupying yourself with activities that can refuel your mood and your physical stamina. Seek out advice from a GAPS practitioner (see page 48) regarding these and other proactive steps.

Getting the Support You Need

Hire a trained GAPS practitioner to handle the details of tailoring the diet to your needs and figuring out the best way to approach your meal planning.

It can be overwhelming when you are diagnosed with GAPS. You feel tired all the time, and now you have to put even *more* time and planning into meal preparation? Yes, it's a lot to take in, but keep in mind that you don't have to do it alone. Hire a trained GAPS practitioner to handle the details of tailoring the diet to your needs and figuring out the best way to approach your meal planning, and rely on social media when you need to ask questions and get encouragement from people who are in the same boat.

GAPS Practitioners

When you're starting the GAPS diet, it is a good idea to get help from a GAPS practitioner, in part to get the relevant tests, in part for professional support and in part to find out from the get-go whether you have specific issues that need to be addressed. A trained GAPS practitioner can help you establish, for example, whether you have problems with candida, histamines, digestion of fat, heavy metals or parasites. Problems like these can bring the healing process to a standstill, which means the diet will be a frustrating experience rather than a success.

Facebook, GAPS Diet Group, August 17, 2015

Claire M
Has anyone suffering from chronic fatigue syndrome experienced an improvement on the GAPS diet?

Sheila H
Yes, the GAPS diet has helped me. Chronic fatigue syndrome derives from inflammation and poisoning, against which the GAPS diet is helpful. If the chronic fatigue persists after a while on the diet, I suggest getting tested to see whether there are any underlying causes, such as Lyme disease, mold fungus or heavy metals. These need to be dealt with through other treatments. In my case, while on the diet, I also needed help with my adrenalin glands and liver due to stress from heavy metals.

My Own GAPS Experience

Although I was vigilant about consulting a professional practitioner on my daughter's behalf, I never bothered to talk to her about my own health. If I had done so, I would probably have been spared a good amount of frustration. It took me a disproportionate amount of time to realize that I, too, had an ailing gut flora, and as a result, I was at a standstill for years.

For the first few years that Karen was on the diet, I supported her by not eating sugar or starch. But it eventually occurred to me that I had not actually been on the GAPS diet all that time, as I thought I had, because I hadn't been drinking bone broth or stock on a daily basis. I was giving all that good stuff to Karen, and I was happy it was helping her, but in my eagerness to help Karen, I had failed to recognize my own need to heal. I had not acknowledged that my own health was worse than I wanted to believe, and I hadn't been tested myself.

For example, I didn't know that I'd been dealing with excess candida for decades. My symptoms included an irritating form of bloat and an inability to get a good night's sleep (the latter can occur because a residual product of candida ultimately prevents the production of sufficient amounts of sleep hormones).

Not until 3 years after Karen began following the GAPS diet did I start trying to get my candida under control by going "all in" on the GAPS diet. It helped, but did 3 years really have to pass for me to get to that point?

Updated lists of professional GAPS practitioners can be found online at www.gaps.me. GAPS is a registered trademark, and you must be a certified GAPS practitioner in order to refer to yourself as such. This guarantees that the practitioners on this list are acquainted with the principles of the GAPS protocol and are able to use them reliably in their professional guidance and recommendations.

Social Media Support

Aside from getting advice from a competent practitioner, there is a lot of help to be found on discussion boards in Facebook and Yahoo! Groups. Even if you are not on Facebook as a matter of principle, you may want to become a member for the sole purpose of participating in these groups. The support they offer is invaluable. You can ask specific questions and get informed answers from people who have experienced the same types of issues, get moral support if you are stuck in a crisis, and share successes, recipes and more. Plus, it's often just nice to be in contact with someone who can relate from personal experience.

There is a lot of help to be found on discussion boards in Facebook and Yahoo! Groups.

PART 2

Welcome to the GAPS Kitchen

Grocery Shopping for the GAPS Diet

You'll need to adjust several habits while on the GAPS diet, including your grocery shopping practices. You may need to get used to looking for food in different areas of the grocery store than you're used to. For example, if you are used to heading straight for the ready-to-eat dinners, crackers and cookies, you'll need to learn to shop the outer aisles for fresh meat and vegetables, and to avoid packaged foods — you want to prepare your own meals from scratch, using real ingredients. Sometimes it's easiest to buy products online, and this may even become a necessity if you cannot find certain foods in even well-stocked grocery stores.

In addition, expect to do a little research: Is there a local farmers' market that sells good-quality organic produce at reasonable prices? Are there any on-farm sales or farm shops nearby? Does anyone in your network know someone who sells a whole or half animal that you can store in the freezer, or who sells raw honey? Where can you pick strawberries that haven't been exposed to pesticides?

Because the GAPS diet recommends certain specialty meats, including organ meats, it's a good idea to become friends with your local butcher. Learn what cuts of meat they typically have on hand and what you might need to special-order. For special orders, ask how long in advance you need to place the order, and plan ahead so you can make sure you have the meat on hand when you need it.

Take it one ingredient and one step at a time. As you get used to the new foods required by the diet and learn how to acquire them easily, your new shopping habits will

Did You Know?

Always Read Labels

A surprising number of the so-called food products available today have been so altered by the industry that they can no longer be considered natural foods. That's why it's so important to be alert when shopping. Bring a magnifying glass so you can check labels. Be critical, and if you don't recognize an ingredient on a label, do some research to find out what it is before purchasing that product.

Choose Organic (and Preferably Local) Foods

Since one of the purposes of the GAPS diet is detoxification, it's important to limit your intake of pesticides, heavy metals, antibiotics and other substances that may contribute to wrecking a healthy gut flora. So choose organic foods whenever possible. If, for financial reasons, you must choose between organic produce or organic meat, then choose organic produce. Vegetables and fruits have no internal cleansing system, as animals do. If you must make choices about which vegetables and fruits to purchase organic and which to save some money on, then visit the Environmental Working Group's website (ewg.org). Every year they publish a list of the "Dirty Dozen" (foods you should definitely purchase organic versions of) and the "Clean Fifteen" (foods with few, if any, pesticide residues).

become routine, and you will able to relax and let your brain concentrate on other things.

Specialty Ingredients

Many of the ingredients you'll need to prepare the recipes in this book are easily found in any supermarket, but in the GAPS diet, we're always looking for the best-quality, freshest ingredients with the least amount of toxins and additives. That means you might have to do some extra work as you make your way through the store. Instead of simply picking up the first package of chicken breasts that catches your eye, you'll want to take your time and make sure the meat you buy comes from free-range chickens. Instead of just grabbing any old vegetable oil, make sure to choose cold-pressed olive oil. Look for tomatoes in glass containers rather than cans, to avoid the chemicals that cans can leach into the food.

In addition, my recipes include some ingredients that may be harder to find, such as tomato vinegar and sesame flour. You may need to visit a health food or specialty food store to find them, or may even need to order them online. I have included these ingredients either because they are a good substitute for a GAPS-unfriendly food item, enabling us to prepare recipes that would otherwise be impossible to enjoy on this diet, or because they deliver so much flavor or health benefits that they are worth the extra effort it takes to track them down.

Below you'll find some more detailed information on some of the specialty ingredients used in this book.

Ethical Meat Products

The GAPS protocol recommends choosing only meat from animals that were raised in a natural habitat and fed food that is natural for their species. For example, chickens should be free-range, cows should be grass-fed, and pigs should be free to work the soil with their snouts.

Ethical treatment of the animals is obviously good for its own sake, but it also means higher-quality meat. To understand why, consider the digestive system of a cow, which is ideally suited for digesting grass. When we replace the cow's natural food with something else, such as soy, the cow cannot digest its food as easily, and that affects the quality of its meat (and the milk it delivers). Such meat is measurably less nourishing than meat from grass-fed cows, which is rich in vital vitamins and minerals.

> **Did You Know?**
>
> **Crowd-Sourcing**
> If you're having trouble finding an ingredient, or are looking for a better or less expensive source, consider posting your question on social media. There is almost always an answer of some kind to be found.

Ethical treatment of the animals is obviously good for its own sake, but it also means higher-quality meat.

Filtered Water

Depending on where you live, you may be lucky enough to have clean drinking water available right from the tap. But if there are high levels of toxins in the tap water in your area — or if you're not sure whether your water is contaminated with toxins or clean — it's a good idea to filter your drinking water and the water you use for cooking your food.

Cold-Pressed Plant Oils

Always choose cold-pressed plant oils, such as olive oil and coconut oil, as cold-pressing keeps the fragile fatty acids in the oils intact. If a plant oil isn't cold-pressed, it is already ruined at the time of purchase.

Raw Honey

Raw honey, also known as cold-slung honey, has an enormous number of nutrients, many of which are heat-sensitive and are therefore destroyed by heat pasteurization. It also has antimicrobial properties. Use it in any recipe that is not heated. For recipes that are heated, you can be less fussy and use any type of honey, as the heat will destroy the nutrients anyway.

Tomato Vinegar

Tomato vinegar adds a pleasant umami flavor to recipes. It's unlikely you'll find it in your local supermarket, but you might have better luck at a gourmet food store. If not, you can order it online. When a recipe calls for tomato vinegar and you don't have any on hand, you can try using a good-quality no-sugar-added balsamic vinegar in its place, keeping in mind that the resulting flavor of the recipe will be different.

Tomatoes in Glass Jars

Instead of buying canned tomatoes, look for tomatoes packed in glass jars. Unlike cans, which may be lined with chemicals that can contaminate the food within, glass is inert. Jars of tomatoes may be a bit harder to find, but it will be worth the added effort to keep unwanted chemicals from entering your body.

In addition, make sure the processed tomatoes you buy are free of added sugar or starch of any kind.

Sesame Flour

Sesame flour is a starch-free flour that is rich in minerals and vitamins. It is available online and at some well-stocked health food stores. If you cannot find it, you can make your own by grinding sesame seeds in your nut grinder (see box, page 75).

Shredded Coconut

Grate a fresh coconut or buy unsweetened coarsely shredded coconut of good quality. It is possible to purchase some inexpensive but very poor-quality shredded coconut; that won't do. If you cannot find high-quality shredded coconut, buy a coconut, wrap it in a towel and crack it open with a hammer (saving the liquid inside, if you can). Pry out the white meat, then use a vegetable peeler to pare off the brown skin. Grate the meat with a box grater or the grating disk of a food processor.

Unflavored Gelatin Powder

Choose a good-quality brand made from grass-fed animals, such as Great Lakes or Vital Protein. Make sure to get the type of gelatin that can congeal and thicken, not the type meant only as a supplement. Look for one with a product description on the package so you can read what it is based on and what it contains.

Balancing Your Budget

Although purchasing organic foods, special-order meats from your butcher and specialty ingredients online can cost a bit more than you might be used to spending on groceries, keep in mind all the expenses you will no longer have: you won't need to buy expensive lean meats anymore, you won't be buying those pricy prepared and processed foods, and there will be no spontaneous visits to the bakery, the hot dog stand or the candy store. You'll be eating very little takeout food and won't dine out all that often. Plus, as you start to feel better, you may no longer need certain medications to treat your symptoms, so you'll see a savings there, too.

Did You Know?

Cheap Out on Meat

When you're on the GAPS diet, you'll be eating a lot of organ meats, along with fattier cuts of meat than you may be used to. That's because lean meat in and of itself, without accompanying fat, does not have a healing effect; effective absorption of meat's nutrients is dependent on the presence of fat. Happily, fatty cuts and organ meats are typically much less expensive than those lean, deboned, trimmed meat cuts, so in addition to getting healthy, you'll be saving money!

Useful Tools in the GAPS Kitchen

Did You Know?

Seek Out Sales

You can often find kitchen tools on sale at a deep discount in secondhand shops or at a local flea market. If all else fails, you can always add them to your wish list for your birthday!

Compared with our great-grandmothers, we have truly remarkable access to kitchen utensils and appliances, including refrigerators and freezers, that can relieve some of the worst strains of kitchen work. The tools listed below are by no means all necessary, but many of them do make life considerably easier than if we were to prepare everything in the same laborious manner as our foremothers.

When considering whether to buy the tools on this list, you may want to ask yourself, "Is this something I really need, or would it just be nice to have?" The answer is individual. There are only two items that I recommend you have on hand right from the start: a proper pot or jar in which to ferment vegetables and a large pot in which to cook stock and bone broth.

The items mentioned below (listed in order of priority) are supplementary to the basic tools that most kitchens should already be equipped with, such as sharp knives, cutting boards, measuring cups and spoons, pots and pans, and lots of mixing bowls in various sizes.

Did You Know?

Why Not Aluminum?

Aluminum leaches into your food if you use aluminum pots and pans for cooking. Since we're trying to keep all toxins, including metals, out of our bodies, it only makes sense to avoid the use of aluminum kitchenware.

- Classic fermentation crock or mason jar with an airlock lid (for making sauerkraut and other fermented vegetables)
- Large pot (not aluminum) that holds $2\frac{1}{2}$ to 3 gallons (10 to 12 L), with a lid (for cooking stock and bone broth)
- Spacious freezer
- Mandoline
- Stomper, also known as a tamper or pounder (for making sauerkraut)
- Food thermometer (for making yogurt and sour cream)
- Mini food processor or spice grinder (for fine grinding)
- Blender or food processor
- Immersion blender (for puréeing soups and sauces)
- Real, old-fashioned whisk
- Long palette knife, also known as a crêpe knife
- Crêpe pan (for making pancakes and omelets)
- Food storage containers in various sizes with tight-sealing lids, suitable for transportation
- Lunch boxes with compartments or individual boxes with cooling elements

- Insulated bottle with a broad mouth (it's easier to wash) for transporting stock and broth
- Funnel and plastic strainer (for making kefir)
- Vegetable peeler or spiralizer (for making vegetable pasta)
- Juicer
- Yogurt maker (yogurt can also be made in the oven)
- Food dehydrator
- Meat grinder
- Slow cooker (for cooking bone broth and other dishes)
- Ice cream maker
- Electric waffle maker

Meal Plans for the GAPS Diet

Now that you are on the GAPS diet and are preparing most of your meals yourself, you will need to plan farther ahead than you may be used to, and that's where meal planning comes in. I've provided 30 days' worth of sample meal plans — 18 days of intro diet meals and 12 days of full GAPS diet meals — to get you going, but bear in mind that these are really just suggestions. Use them for inspiration and refer to the "What to Eat" lists on pages 21–23 (for the intro diet) and 30–32 (for the full GAPS diet) to create customized meals according to your own preferences and specialized needs, such as any food intolerances.

Remember not to rush through the various stages of the intro diet; move through them at your own pace. I have provided 3 days' worth of meal plans per stage, but the amount of time you will actually need to spend in each stage is very individual, so repeat the meals (or mix them up) as needed. In each stage, you can also continue to eat any of the meals mentioned in the previous stage. Also keep in mind that, although your food options may be limited during the first stages of the intro diet, this is not a starvation diet. Eat as often and as much of the available options as you please.

Welcome to the world of the GAPS kitchen, filled with delicious, high-quality food as your great-grandmother might (almost) have made it. I hope that my meal plans, and the recipes that follow in part 3, will inspire you and support you on your GAPS journey to a healthy life, free of symptoms!

Did You Know?

Nuts and Seeds

Nuts and large seeds, such as pumpkin and sunflower seeds, must be soaked and dried as directed on page 74 before you eat them or incorporate them into a recipe.

Did You Know?

Fermented Foods

Take it slow with fermented foods, such as sauerkraut brine and whey: start with small amounts and increase gradually. See "How to Increase Your Intake of Probiotics" (page 28) for more information.

Intro Diet, Stage 1

	Day 1	Day 2	Day 3
Breakfast and Snacks	Chicken Stock (page 102) with some of the meat and skin, well-cooked vegetables and sauerkraut brine	Veal Stock (page 102) or other meat stock with tomatoes and sauerkraut brine	Mediterranean Stock (page 107)
Lunch	Fish Stock (page 103) with some of the fish, well-cooked vegetables and sauerkraut brine	Cauliflower Chicken Stock (page 106) Baked Pumpkin or Squash (page 77)	Fish Stock with Shrimp (page 105) with green peas or other well-cooked vegetables and sauerkraut brine
Dinner	Beef Vegetable Soup (page 110) Baked Pumpkin or Squash (page 77)	Fish Stock (page 103) with some of the fish, well-cooked vegetables and sauerkraut brine	Veal Stock (page 102) or other meat stock with tomatoes and sauerkraut brine Baked Pumpkin or Squash (page 77)
Beverages	Filtered water Sparkling water Vallentino's Favorite Drink (page 206) Herbal teas, such as Chamomile Tea or Ginger Tea (page 205) with a little honey		

Intro Diet, Stage 2

	Day 1	Day 2	Day 3
Breakfast	Stock with Poached Egg (page 104), made with egg yolk, with added well-cooked vegetables and sauerkraut brine	Stock with Poached Egg (page 104) with added well-cooked vegetables and sauerkraut brine	Stock with Poached Egg (page 104) with added well-cooked vegetables and sauerkraut brine
Lunch	Cauliflower Chicken Stock (page 106) Mashed Root Vegetables (page 181)	Gravlax (page 121) Soft-boiled egg Fish Stock (page 103) with added sauerkraut brine	Gravlax (page 121) Fish Soup with Fennel (page 108) with added sauerkraut brine
Dinner	Veal Stew (page 144) Well-cooked vegetables	Hearty Chicken Stew (page 142) Mashed Root Vegetables (page 181)	Meatball Stew with Spinach and Celery Root (page 146)
Snacks	Yogurt (page 92) Ginger Drops (page 257)		
Beverages	As in stage 1		

Intro Diet, Stage 3

	Day 1	Day 2	Day 3
Breakfast	Eggs scrambled with well-cooked vegetables	Zucchini Pancakes (page 119) Well-cooked vegetables	Sour Cream Pancakes (page 217) with Yogurt (page 92) and a dash of honey
Lunch	Lumpfish Roe with Avocado (page 122) Fish Soup with Fennel (page 108)	Chicken Liver Pâté (page 125) Tomato Soup (variation, page 113)	Lunch Wraps with Chicken Filling for Stage 3 (variation, page 115)
Dinner	Turkey, Mushroom and Spinach Stew (page 143)	Corned Tongue in Mushroom Sauce (page 162) Creamed Celery Root (page 175)	Lamb and Cabbage Stew (page 145)
Snacks	**As in stage 2, plus:** Sauerkraut (page 84 or 86)		
Beverages	**As in stage 1, plus:** Kefir (page 94) Stock (page 102 or 103)		

Intro Diet, Stage 4

	Day 1	Day 2	Day 3
Breakfast	Scrambled eggs Nut and Seed Bread (page 270) with butter	Sour Cream Pancakes (page 217) with Yogurt (page 92)	Spinach Pancakes (page 118) with Yogurt (page 92)
Lunch	Fish Cakes (variation, page 151) with Rémoulade (page 189) Cold well-cooked vegetables with Oil and Vinegar Dressing (page 192)	GAPS-Friendly Pizza with a Crispy Crust (page 160; see tip)	Beef or Veal Liver Pâté (variation, page 126) Cauliflower Soup (variation, page 111) Nut and Seed Bread (page 270)
Dinner	Baked Salmon (variation, page 149) White Asparagus with Lemon Butter (variation, page 171)	Carrot and Zucchini Spaghetti (page 182) with Bolognese Sauce (page 158) Italian Salad (page 133)	Slow-Braised Pork Hocks (page 156) Oven-Baked Vegetables (variation, page 180)
Snacks	**As in stage 3, plus:** Olives Nuts (page 74) Salted Almonds (page 201)	Almond and Seed Crackers (page 200) Beet Chips (page 198)	Sesame Crisps (page 199) Guacamole (variation, page 139)
Beverages	**As in stage 3, plus:** GAPS Smoothie (page 209)	Carrot Juice (page 206), with or without added whey	Green Juice (page 207)

Intro Diet, Stage 5

	Day 1	Day 2	Day 3
Breakfast	Scrambled eggs Nut and Seed Bread (page 270) with butter Yogurt (page 92)	GAPS Smoothie (page 209) Nut and Seed Bread (page 270) with butter	Scrambled eggs Tomatoes and cucumber slices with Sour Cream (page 92)
Lunch	Lunch Wraps with Salmon Filling (page 114)	Cold corned tongue leftovers Sauerkraut (page 84 or 86) Italian Salad (page 133)	GAPS Sushi (page 123) Nut and Seed Bread (page 270) with butter
Dinner	Corned Tongue in Mushroom Sauce (page 162) Mashed Root Vegetables (page 181)	Meatballs (page 157) Sweet-and-Sour Red Cabbage (page 172) Root Vegetable Patties (page 136)	Apple Pork (page 154) Sauerkraut (page 84 or 86) Oven-Baked Vegetables (variation, page 180)
Snacks	**As in stage 4, plus:** Carrot sticks Cucumber slices Cherry tomatoes Applesauce (page 219) Marinated Sun-Dried Tomatoes (page 197)		
Beverages	**As in stage 4, plus:** Carrot, Apple and Celery Juice (page 208), with or without added whey		

Intro Diet, Stage 6

	Day 1	Day 2	Day 3
Breakfast	Banana Pancakes (page 216) with berries and Yogurt (page 92)	Sour Cream Pancakes (page 217) with Applesauce (page 219)	Soft-boiled egg Nut and Seed Bread (page 270) with butter
Lunch	GAPS-Friendly Pizza with a Crispy Crust (page 160; see tip) Brussels Sprout and Apple Salad (page 135)	Lamb Liver Pâté (page 128) Nut and Seed Bread (page 270) Italian Salad (page 133)	Vitello Tornado (page 130) Green salad with grated carrots and Oil and Vinegar Dressing (page 192)
Dinner	Baked Salmon (page 149) with Ravigote Sauce (page 189) White Asparagus with Lemon Butter (page 171)	Sweet-and-Sour Pork (page 155) Sauerkraut (page 84 or 86) Cauliflower Couscous (page 174)	Fried Liver with Onions and Mushrooms (page 159) Creamed Celery Root (page 175)
Snacks	**As in stage 5, plus:** Brazil nuts (soaked and dried) Dried fruit Banana Bread (page 271) Tarte Tatin à la GAPS (page 238) Almond Tuiles (page 252) Quick Strawberry Ice Cream (page 232) Berry Iced Kefir (page 232)		
Beverages	**As in stage 5, plus:** Filtered water with lemon slice Sparkling water with lemon slice Unsweetened nonalcoholic fruit cider Lemon Tea (page 205) Kefir Eggnog (page 211) Carrot and Avocado Smoothie (page 210), with or without added whey		

Full GAPS Diet

- Instead of stock, drink Bone Broth (page 99) and Fish Bone Broth (page 101) daily, as many times as you like throughout the day.

- Eat probiotic foods like Sauerkraut (page 84 or 86), Yogurt or Sour Cream (page 92) and Kefir (page 94) often. Add sauerkraut brine, yogurt whey or kefir whey to broths and soups. Whey also makes a great addition to juices and smoothies.

- **Snacks:** In addition to the options mentioned in the intro diet meal plans, enjoy raw coconut, aged hard cheese, blue cheese, red culture cheese or white cheese, and any of the snacks (pages 196–201) or sweets (pages 216–267) in the book.

- **Beverages:** Enjoy any of the options on the "What to Eat" lists (pages 30–32) and in the Beverages chapter (page 204–213).

	Day 1	Day 2	Day 3
Breakfast	Pizza Omelet (page 116) Freshly pressed juice	Yogurt (page 92) with nuts, grated coconut and fresh fruit Freshly pressed juice	Eggs scrambled with roasted vegetables Freshly pressed juice
Lunch	Chicken Nuggets (page 131) with Peanut Butter Sauce (page 185) Cucumber Mint Salad (page 136)	Smiling Eggs with Mustard Mayo (page 117) Kimchi (page 88) with Sour Cream (page 92)	Lunch Wraps with Ham and Cheese Filling (page 114) Green salad with Oil and Vinegar Dressing (page 192)
Dinner	Veal Tails in Red Wine (page 165) Root Vegetable Patties (page 136)	Fish Fillets with Spinach (page 150) Cauliflower Gratin (page 173)	Lamb Meatballs in Spicy Tomato Sauce (page 167) Leeks au Gratin (page 175)

	Day 4	Day 5	Day 6
Breakfast	Yogurt (page 92) with nuts, grated coconut and berries Freshly pressed juice	Bacon and eggs Tomato Salsa (page 87) Freshly pressed juice	Yogurt (page 92) with nuts, grated coconut and banana Freshly pressed juice
Lunch	Beef or Veal Liver Pâté (page 126) with Jellied Broth (page 193) Beet Salad (page 134)	Hokkaido Squash Soup (page 112) Spinach Pie (page 178)	Shrimp Bisque (page 109) Nut and Seed Bread (page 270) with blue cheese
Dinner	Oven-Baked Mackerel with Apple Compote (page 147) Mushrooms with Spinach (page 177)	Thai-Style Chicken Legs (page 153) Cauliflower Couscous (page 174)	Stuffed Portobello Mushrooms (page 176) Bone Broth with Poached Egg (variation, page 104)

	Day 7	Day 8	Day 9
Breakfast	Yogurt (page 92) with almonds, grated coconut, apples and raisins Freshly pressed juice	Sour Cream Pancakes (page 217) with berries Freshly pressed juice	Yogurt (page 92) with nuts, seeds and grated coconut Freshly pressed juice
Lunch	Jazzed-Up Shrimp (page 124) White Bean Hummus (page 139) with olives and carrot sticks	Club Salad (page 132) Nut and Seed Bread (page 270) with butter	Lunch Wraps with Chicken Filling (page 114)
Dinner	Osso Buco (page 164) Mashed Root Vegetables (page 181)	Carrot and Zucchini Spaghetti (page 182) with Meatballs (page 157), tomatoes and Pesto (page 191)	Lamb-Stuffed Spinach Pancakes (page 168) with Tomato Salsa (page 87)
	Day 10	Day 11	Day 12
Breakfast	Soft-boiled egg Nut and Seed Bread (page 270) with butter Carrot and Avocado Smoothie (page 210)	Zucchini Pancakes (page 119) with tomatoes and mushrooms Freshly pressed juice	Yogurt (page 92) with nuts, grated coconut and banana Freshly pressed juice
Lunch	Fish Cakes (page 151) with Aïoli (page 188) and Soft-Curd Cheese with Herbs (page 196)	Lamb Liver Pâté (page 128) Cucumber Mint Salad (page 136)	Falafels (page 138) Spicy Soft-Curd Cheese (page 196)
Dinner	Sweet-and-Sour Pork (page 155) Kimchi (page 88) Oven-Baked Vegetables (page 180)	Fish Lasagna (page 152) Green salad with nuts and Oil and Vinegar Dressing (page 192)	T-bone steak served with Béarnaise Sauce (page 186) Beet Salad (page 134)

PART 3

Recipes for the GAPS Diet

The Recipe Tags

All of the recipes are accompanied by a tag that indicates when it is safe for you to start enjoying them. For example, if a recipe tag says "Intro Diet, Stage 4," that means you can eat it once you have reached stage 4 of the intro diet. But, of course, you can continue enjoying the recipe once you have progressed into stages 5 and 6, as well as while you're on the full GAPS diet and beyond! Recipes that you can experiment with once you are ready to transition out of the GAPS diet are labeled "Transition Diet."

You'll find a list of the recipes that are suitable for the intro diet on pages 24–25.

Staples in the GAPS Kitchen

In addition to fermented foods, for which recipes follow in the next chapter, there are several other types of prepared foods and flavorings that can be very useful to have on hand in the cupboard, refrigerator or freezer, to use when needed. The recipes in this chapter will allow you to prepare GAPS-friendly ingredients in advance for use at a moment's notice. Remember, you can take your time when preparing your initial batches of these items — you don't need to make everything all at once! Just prepare one ingredient at a time, and when you see that you are about to run out of something, make a new batch when you have time.

Clarified Butter

**Makes about
1¾ cups (425 mL)**

If you are lactose-intolerant, try clarifying butter for use in cooking. Most people are able to tolerate clarified butter from the very beginning of the GAPS diet, but experiment carefully.

Tips

The smoking point for butter is 354°F (177°C); for clarified butter, it is as high as 485°F (252°C). This makes it easier to work with clarified butter (nobody wants burnt butter).

Many Gapsters use the word "ghee" interchangeably with "clarified butter." However, while ghee is an Indian type of clarified butter, it is made using a different process.

- **Preheat oven to 200°F (100°C), with rack set in the second-lowest position**
- **Loaf pan (preferably made of stone or clay)**

| 1 lb | butter | 500 g |

1. Add butter to the loaf pan and place the pan in the preheated oven. Cook for about 30 minutes or until butter is melted and has separated into two layers: a white bottom layer covered by clear yellow fat.

2. Carefully pour the clarified fat into a large airtight container, making sure to keep the white layer separate. You can use a spoon to skim off the last bit of clarified butter. Discard the white sediment. Store the clarified butter in the refrigerator for up to 6 months.

Flaxseed Egg Substitute

1²⁄₃ oz	flax seeds	50 g
2 cups	water	500 mL

**Makes 2 cups
(500 mL)**

If you cannot tolerate eggs, you can use this substitute in recipes where eggs are typically used to bind ingredients together, such as when making ground meat mixtures (for meatballs, for example), fish cakes, pizza crusts or baked goods. Do note, however, that this substitute cannot be whisked.

Tips

Use 3 tbsp (45 mL) flaxseed egg substitute to replace each egg in your recipe.

You can use the boiled seeds to make Almond and Seed Crackers (page 200) or Nut Seed Bread (page 270).

1. Place seeds and water in a saucepan and bring to a boil over high heat. Continue boiling, stirring constantly, for 5 minutes.

2. Strain the liquid through a fine-mesh sieve into an airtight container and either discard the seeds or keep them for another use (see tip). Let cool, then store in the refrigerator for up to 1 week.

Duck or Goose Fat

**Makes about
8 oz (250 g)**

*Never skimp on good fat
while on the GAPS diet.
Reserve any fat you don't
eat from poultry, lamb,
veal, pork or beef. You
can either melt it and use
it in cooking, or reserve
it for making Bone Broth
(page 99), adding it with
the bones in step 2. To get
a big enough portion of fat
to last for several months,
it makes sense to roast
fatty poultry, like duck or
goose, to collect the fat
rendered during roasting.
As a bonus, once you are
in stage 4, you end up
with a roast that will taste
wonderful served with
vegetables and gravy.*

Tips

Most of the fat rendered
from poultry consists of
monounsaturated fatty
acids, so it liquefies at
room temperature.

Duck or goose fat is a
natural choice for frying or
sautéing when you want
the extra-deep flavor it
adds to a dish.

- *Preheat oven to 325°F (160°C)*
- *Roasting pan*

7 lb	duck or goose	3.5 kg
3 tbsp	salt, divided	45 mL
½ cup	water	125 mL

1. Place duck or goose in roasting pan and sprinkle all over with 1 tbsp (15 mL) salt (adding salt sparsely in the beginning ensures that the fat rendered doesn't get too salty). Roast in preheated oven for 1 hour.

2. Remove duck from oven and pour off as much fat as possible into a large bowl. Let cool.

3. Sprinkle duck with the remaining salt, add water to the pan and continue roasting for 2 hours or until an instant-read thermometer inserted in the thickest part of a thigh registers 165°F (74°C). (To give the duck a crispy golden brown color and improve the flavor, increase the oven temperature to 480°F/250°C for the last 15 minutes of roasting.) Carve and serve or store the meat as desired.

4. Divide the cooled fat into smaller portions and store in airtight containers in the refrigerator for up to 1 month or in the freezer for up to 1 year. Use a sharp knife to cut off a slice of the cold or frozen fat as needed.

Soft-Curd Cheese

**Makes about
5 oz (150 g)**

*Once some healing has
taken place and you can
tolerate fermented milk,
it's nice to have ready-to-
use soft-curd cheese in
the fridge. Serve it with
breakfast, lunch or supper,
or as a snack. Mix it with
herbs or spices and use it as
a condiment or as a filling
in a wrap. If you feel like a
little sweet something, just
mix it with a dash of raw
honey and enjoy.*

Tip
See recipes for Soft-Curd
Cheese with Herbs and Spicy
Soft-Curd Cheese (page 196).

- *Strainer lined with a clean, tightly woven, lint-free tea towel*

4 cups	Kefir (page 94)	1 L

1. Pour kefir into prepared strainer and let the whey drain off for 24 hours in a cool place. Save the whey for another use (see tip, page 95).

2. After draining, the soft-curd cheese remains as a soft, creamy substance. Store in an airtight container in the refrigerator for up to 1 week.

White Beans and Lima Beans

Makes about 11 cups (2.75 L)

For Gapsters' consumption, white beans and lima beans must be extremely tender. We are talking 4 to 6 hours of cooking — much, much longer than the instructions on the package of dried beans. Prepare a large amount at a time and store the cooked beans in smaller portions.

Tips

Use whole beans in stews and salads; use mashed beans to make minced meat or a gratin. White beans can easily substitute for chickpeas in hummus or for kidney beans in chili.

Wait to add salt until the very end of the cooking process. If it is added at the beginning, the beans will become strangely chewy.

2 lbs	dried navy beans, Great Northern beans, baby lima beans or lima beans	1 kg
	Cold water	
	Salt (see tip)	

1. Pour beans into a large bowl and cover with plenty of cold water. Cover loosely and let soak at room temperature for 24 to 48 hours, rinsing them several times and recovering with fresh cold water.

2. Drain off water, transfer beans to a pot and cover with plenty of fresh cold water. Remove any shells that have loosened from beans. Bring to a boil over high heat. Skim water, reduce heat and simmer for 4 to 6 hours or until beans are extremely tender and mash easily. Add a small amount of salt and simmer for 5 minutes.

3. Drain and rinse beans. Serve immediately or let cool, then transfer to airtight containers and store in the freezer for up to 6 months. Thaw overnight in the refrigerator before use, or add frozen to the dish you are cooking and cook until heated through.

More Bean Tips

- Consider introducing beans only after all digestive symptoms are gone. Even after proper preparation, some people may find beans difficult or impossible to digest.
- White beans (except cannellini beans, also known as white kidney beans), lima beans, split peas and lentils (see page 73) are the only legumes that are GAPS-friendly — and only if they are correctly prepared, as in these recipes.
- Store-bought flours made from dried beans or lentils are not recommended during the GAPS diet, as the beans have not undergone this pretreatment.
- According to *Nourishing Traditions* by Sally Fallon and Mary G. Enig, our ancestors also soaked and cooked dried legumes for a long time.

Lentils and Split Peas

**Makes about
15 cups (3.75 L)**

2 lbs	dried red, brown, green or yellow lentils or split peas, rinsed	1 kg
	Cold water	
	Bone Broth (page 99; optional)	
Pinch	salt (see tip)	Pinch

Like dried beans (see page 72), lentils and split peas must be soaked and cooked quite a bit longer than is indicated on the package before Gapsters can enjoy them. Prepare a large batch at a time and freeze the cooked lentils or split peas in smaller portions.

1. Pour lentils or split peas into a large bowl and cover with plenty of cold water. Cover loosely and let soak at room temperature for 12 to 48 hours, rinsing them several times and recovering with fresh cold water.

2. Drain off water, transfer lentils or split peas to a pot and cover with plenty of bone broth or fresh cold water. Bring to a boil over high heat. Skim liquid, reduce heat and simmer for 1 hour. Add a small amount of salt and simmer for 5 minutes.

3. Drain and rinse lentils or split peas. Serve immediately or let cool, then transfer to airtight containers and store in the freezer for up to 6 months. Thaw overnight in the refrigerator before use, or add frozen to the dish you are cooking and cook until heated through.

Tips

If you're adding lentils or split peas to a soup or stew, you can soak them as in step 1, then add them directly to the pot, but the soup or stew must then be cooked for at least 1 hour.

Wait to add salt until the very end of the cooking process. If it is added at the beginning, the lentils or split peas will become strangely chewy.

More Lentil and Split Pea Tips

- Consider introducing lentils and split peas only after all digestive symptoms are gone. Even after proper preparation, some people may find lentils and split peas difficult or impossible to digest.

- Red lentils tend to boil to mush and are suited for soups such as the spicy Indian soup dahl. They can also be added to pâté, minced meat or mashed root vegetables to stretch the dish, or can add more substance to a gratin.

- Brown lentils and green lentils, like de Puy, Pardina or Beluga (which look closer to black), don't turn to mush as easily as red lentils and are good in dishes made with lamb, duck or game.

- Yellow lentils are good with pork or as a substitute for peas in split pea soup.

- Split peas tend to get mushy and are therefore useful for thickening a soup or sauce. They are also good in casseroles with pork or lamb.

Nuts and Seeds

Makes about 9 oz (270 g)

It can be difficult for a weak gut to digest nuts and larger seeds, such as pumpkin and sunflower seeds. Soaking them in salt water for 12 hours first can make it a lot easier — for some people, it makes all the difference in their ability to tolerate nuts and seeds.

Tips

Wait to eat Brazil nuts and pistachios until stage 6, as they may contain a higher level of toxins than other nuts.

After going through this process, nuts and seeds become more fragile and must be used within 4 to 6 days if stored at room temperature. They may be kept in the refrigerator for up to 3 weeks or in the freezer for up to 3 months.

- • *Electric dehydrator (optional)*

10 oz	nuts or seeds	300 g
2 tbsp	salt	30 mL
4 cups	cold water	1 L

1. Add nuts, salt and water to a large bowl and let soak at room temperature for 12 hours.

2. Drain off water. Rinse nuts thoroughly in cold water three times, then pat nuts dry.

3. Spread nuts onto mesh drying racks or baking sheets (for oven-drying). Dry nuts in a dehydrator or in the oven at 150°F (65°C) for 1 to 3 hours or until very crunchy.

Blanching Almonds

To blanch almonds, bring 4 cups (1 L) water to a boil and add 1 cup (250 mL) dried soaked almonds. Return to a boil and cook for 10 to 30 seconds or until almond skins are loose. Drain off water, sprinkle almonds with cold water, and peel off skins.

Toasting Nuts and Seeds

Heat a dry skillet over medium heat. Spread dried soaked nuts or seeds into a single layer in the pan and cook, stirring often to avoid burning, for 3 to 4 minutes or until golden brown. Immediately transfer nuts or seeds to a plate, spread out in a single layer and let cool.

  If toasting chopped nuts, keep in mind that small pieces can get semi-burnt before the bigger pieces turn golden. When the small pieces are nicely toasted, remove them by sifting them through a coarse strainer, then finish toasting the remaining big pieces.

Finely Chopping Nuts

When a recipe calls for finely chopped nuts, chop them by hand with a sharp knife, as it can be difficult to do in a nut grinder — before you know it, you have nut flour instead of chopped nuts. You are aiming for pieces that are the size of a half or whole grain of corn (though it's very much a matter of preference).

Tips

When they are dehydrated as in step 3, the weight of nuts and seeds decreases by about 10%.

I only blanch almonds (remove the skins) for special occasions; otherwise, it is not necessary. I sometimes peel off any loose skin from hazelnuts once they are soaked and dried.

Making Nut or Seed Flour

To grind dried soaked nuts or seeds into flour, add them to your nut grinder (see below) and pulse until the flour is the desired consistency. This can happen very fast, depending on your equipment. Stop before the flour becomes buttery.

Many of the recipes in this book ask you to grind nuts or seeds to a particular consistency. Here's what I mean by fine or medium-fine flour:

- *Fine flour* has grains about the size of coarse yellow cornmeal.
- *Medium-fine flour* has grains slightly larger than coarse raw cane sugar.

For optimum freshness, wait to grind nuts and seeds into flour until you need the flour for a recipe. If you decide to grind a bigger batch of flour than you need for your recipe, store it in the refrigerator for up to 2 weeks or in the freezer for up to 3 months.

Nut Grinders

There are several different tools you can use to grind nuts and seeds, including a food processor, a high-powered blender (such as a Vitamix) or, for small amounts, a mini food processor, a mini chopper attachment for an immersion blender or a spice or coffee grinder.

Coconut Milk

**Makes about 2 cups
(500 mL)**

*Coconut milk is good in
lots of recipes, from soups
to ice cream. But quality
is key! If you can't find
organic coconut milk
with no additives, make
your own coconut milk
instead, using good-quality
coarsely shredded coconut.*

Tips

Coconut milk separates
when cold. That may be
advantageous if you are
planning to make Coconut
Whipped Cream (page 261).
Otherwise, you can whisk it
back together.

The next best solution if
you can't make your own is
buying organic coconut milk
without any additives.

- *Blender*
- *Strainer lined with cheesecloth or a nut milk bag*

1¼ cups	unsweetened coarsely shredded coconut	300 mL
2½ cups	boiling water	625 mL

1. Place coconut in a large bowl and pour in boiling water. Let stand for 20 minutes.

2. Transfer coconut mixture to blender and blend until creamed.

3. Strain milk through the lined strainer and discard coconut fibers (or dry them to use in baked goods).

4. Store coconut milk in an airtight container in the refrigerator for up to 3 days or in the freezer for up to 3 months.

Baked Pumpkin or Squash

INTRO DIET, STAGE 1

Makes about 2¾ cups (675 mL)

Baked pumpkin or squash can be used to make Pumpkin Blinis (page 120) or a quick Hokkaido Squash Soup (page 112). It's also a good filler in casseroles and Fish Cakes (page 151), and, of course, it's essential in Ginger Pumpkin Pie (page 236). Or invent your own mash by mixing it with sour cream and your favorite herbs and spices!

Tips

It may prove practical to make a large batch all at once and freeze it in smaller portions. Bake as many pumpkins or squash as can fit on a baking sheet in the oven.

All kinds of pumpkins and squash work in this recipe. Two of my favorites are butternut and Hokkaido squash.

- *Preheat oven to 400°F (200°C), with rack set in the second-lowest position*
- *Baking sheet, lined with parchment paper*

2 lb	pumpkin or winter squash	1 kg

1. Place pumpkin on prepared baking sheet and bake in preheated oven for about 1 hour or until fork-tender. Let cool for about 30 minutes.

2. Cut pumpkin in half lengthwise and remove seeds with a spoon. Scoop out the flesh from the shell, discarding the shell. Use immediately or transfer pumpkin flesh to airtight containers and store in the freezer for up to 6 months. Let thaw at room temperature or overnight in the refrigerator.

Flavored Honey

**Makes 1 cup
(250 mL)**

Flavored honeys are nice to have on hand for those times when you want to sweeten your yogurt or pancakes. Leave the flavoring in the bottle until all the honey has been enjoyed.

Tips

Use a bit of the honey first to make room for the flavoring.

You can use vanilla beans left over from another recipe if you dry them first (see tip, page 79).

Dried orange peel can also be used in place of the fresh rind.

It is difficult to know how strong a particular chile pepper is. Taste the infused honey and add more chile pepper if you need to intensify the flavor.

Wait to enjoy chile peppers until you are well into the GAPS diet and your stomach isn't too sensitive.

Vanilla Honey

2	vanilla beans	2
1	bottle (8 oz/250 mL) liquid honey (see tip)	1

1. Cut vanilla beans lengthwise into small pieces. Push the pieces into the honey bottle, cover and let steep for at least 1 week before use.

Anise Honey

8	star anise pods, cut in half	8
1	bottle (8 oz/250 mL) liquid honey	1

1. Push star anise into the honey bottle, cover and let steep for at least 1 week before use.

Orange Honey

1	organic orange	1
1	bottle (8 oz/250 mL) liquid honey	1

1. Using a vegetable peeler, peel off strips of orange rind. Carefully insert strips into the honey bottle, cover and let steep for at least 1 week before use. Save the rest of the orange for another use.

Chile Honey

2	small chile peppers (either fresh or dried)	2
1	bottle (8 oz/250 mL) liquid honey	1

1. Cut chiles lengthwise and remove seeds. Push chiles into the honey bottle, cover and let steep for at least 1 week before use.

Vanilla Vodka

6	vanilla beans	6
1	bottle (24 oz/750 mL) vodka	1

**Makes 3 cups
(750 mL)**

Vanilla vodka can be used as an economical substitute in any recipe that calls for vanilla extract. Vanilla extract may contain additives that are not suitable for the GAPS diet; if you do use it, make sure to use only pure vanilla extract, and read the label to make sure it contains only vanilla, water and alcohol, with no other additives.

Tips

Start a new bottle well before the old bottle is empty, so you always have some on hand.

The used vanilla beans can be spread out on a plate to dry, then reused as desired; they still retain flavor.

1. Cut vanilla beans lengthwise and place them in the bottle of vodka. Store in a cool place, rotating the bottle occasionally, for about 2 months before use.

Fermented Foods

Though now modern once again, fermentation is an ancient craft. Fermented foods offer many benefits, including:

1. **Increased shelf life.** Fermentation preserves vegetables, making them last considerably longer than fresh produce.

2. **Improved taste and consistency.** As foods ferment, their flavor becomes deeper and more nuanced, and in many cases their consistency becomes more delicate.

3. **Contribution to a healthy gut flora.** Many fermented foods contain microbes that are beneficial to the digestive system. The GAPS diet includes plenty of sauerkraut, yogurt and kefir, precisely because these filling, tasty and nutritious foods contribute to a healthy gut flora.

Fermenting Vegetables

All across the globe, fermenting fresh, local vegetables has been a common practice for many, many years, and every country has its own specialties. Here, I've provided recipes for some of the most versatile fermented vegetables, which will be useful in any GAPS kitchen: sauerkraut, kimchi and tomato salsa.

About Sauerkraut

Sauerkraut is the mother of all fermented vegetables. When you preserve cabbage by fermenting it in a jar with an airlock lid, it becomes chock-full of probiotics and C vitamins. Humans have known for centuries that fermenting cabbage gives it a longer shelf life and makes it tastier, *and* that it helps us avoid vitamin deficiencies, such as scurvy.

Experience has also proven that *how* we produce sauerkraut is a crucial component of its quality. This observation led to the invention of the fermentation crock, a container that provides ventilation during the fermenting process. In more recent times, we've developed airlock systems that fit mason jars, enabling them to provide the same favorable conditions for successful fermenting as a fermentation crock.

Oxygen-Free Fermentation

There is a difference between fermentation and oxygen-free fermentation. The latter has an enhanced medicinal effect because it contains the highest possible number of beneficial microbes. So oxygen-free fermentation is the method of choice in the GAPS kitchen.

To ferment vegetables in an oxygen-free environment, you need a container with a ventilation system. There are a couple of choices available on the market today:

1. **A fermentation crock.** The design of this traditional German container for sauerkraut is simple: a water seal is used as an airlock, allowing pressure to slip out without letting oxygen in. A fermentation crock also has the advantage of being made of ceramic, preventing light from getting to the cabbage, which should ferment in darkness. Sizes range from 2 to 30 quarts (or liters).

Salt Quantities

When making sauerkraut, you will need to add an amount of salt that corresponds to 2% of the weight of the cabbage, so it's important to have a good kitchen scale. If you want to ferment other vegetables, be aware that the quantity of salt needed will vary. For example, onions and carrots require 2% salt; cucumbers and peppers require 4% to 5% salt; and pepper mixtures that have been mashed or processed in a blender require 10% salt.

2. A mason jar with an airlock lid. Airlock lids have the advantage of fitting mason jars in a variety of sizes. The disadvantage is that the airlock consists of several small parts that can easily get lost and that must be thoroughly rinsed. Airlocks may seem expensive until you compare them to the price of the probiotics you will no longer need to purchase thanks to your excellent homemade sauerkraut. Start with one or two airlocks; you can always get more.

The problem with using an ordinary glass jar or mason jar is that the pressure that develops as carbon dioxide is created during the fermentation process cannot be expelled without the risk of oxygen seeping in. And that is precisely what shouldn't happen in the first 72 hours. During that time, the harmful bacteria and yeasts die because they are not getting any oxygen, while the beneficial bacteria multiply at a high rate because they thrive without oxygen. If even the tiniest bit of oxygen slips into the jar, the chance of mold growing increases.

But why not just let pressure be pressure and avoid lifting the lid for the first 3 days? Because doing so will ruin your chances of getting the best possible medicinal effect from the fermentation. High pressure inhibits the development of beneficial bacteria. The vegetables may still be fermented, but the amount of probiotics will be low in relation to what it could have been if the carbon dioxide had been given the opportunity to diffuse occasionally during the process. (Incidentally, it has been observed that beneficial microbes change their shape when exposed to pressure. The extent to which this affects us when we eat them is unknown.) High pressure can also make the jar explode, which not only makes a big mess, but is also a waste of food and work.

If you compare batches of sauerkraut produced in jars with and without an airlock, the difference is striking. The cabbage fermented in a jar with an airlock not only tastes better, it is also juicier and more tender, and it lasts longer. If you doubt this, try it for yourself!

Did You Know?

Dealing with Mold

If there is mold in your fermented vegetables, it is no use just removing the visible mold. The entire contents of the jar must be thrown out. Food that contains even traces of mold can make you sick.

Making Cold-Water Brine

If you need cold-water brine with a 2% salt concentration to top up the brine level in your jar, here's how to make it. For each 1 quart (1 L) water, bring to a boil and stir in 0.7 oz (20 g) salt until dissolved. Let cool, then chill until cold. For a 3% brine, use 1 oz (30 g) salt. For a 5% brine, use 1.8 oz (53 g) salt.

Sauerkraut in a Fermentation Crock

Makes about 20 cups (5 L)

If you want to make large amounts of sauerkraut at once, use a fermentation crock. When it's fermented, you can easily divide it into several smaller containers, so you won't "disturb" the whole amount every time you want to eat some. Each time you open the lid, there is a risk of harmful microbes gaining access; storage in small containers helps prevent spoilage of the entire batch.

Tips

Fermentation crocks come with a tamper and two semicircular stones that are used to weigh the cabbage down and keep it beneath the brine.

Be exact when adding salt. Too little may result in slimy cabbage, too much may stop the fermentation. To calculate the quantity of salt you need, weigh the trimmed cabbage in ounces or grams and multiply the weight by 0.02; the resulting number is the weight of salt in ounces or grams you should use.

- *Mandoline*
- *5-quart (5 L) fermentation crock (see tip)*

11 lbs	cabbage	5 kg
3½ oz	pure sea salt or Himalayan salt (approx.)	100 g
	Boiling water	
	Cold-water brine (2% salt), if needed	

1. Rinse outer leaves of cabbage thoroughly to remove all dirt. Remove stem and weigh the remaining cabbage to determine the exact amount of salt required (see tip).

2. Using a mandoline, cut cabbage into very thin strips. Cut the last bits into thin strips with a sharp knife.

3. Place cabbage strips in your largest bowl or a clean, sterilized bucket. Sprinkle with the measured salt so it can start macerating.

4. Wash and sterilize the fermentation crock, tamper and stones with boiling water.

5. Transfer cabbage to the fermentation crock and smash it as much as possible with the tamper so it is packed down tightly and is macerating. You should end up with tamped cabbage all the way up to the neck of the container, and the cabbage should be covered with brine. If any cabbage is above the brine, add enough cold-water brine to cover.

6. Place the two stones on top of the cabbage, put the lid on and pour water into the water lock. Store crock at about 68°F (20°C) for 8 to 10 days, then move it to a cooler place, preferably at 59°F (15°C), for 11 to 13 days (3 weeks total).

7. Distribute sauerkraut into clean, sterilized mason jars, making sure it is covered with brine, seal with lids and store in a cool, dark place.

Tips

The cabbage must ferment for 3 weeks total, but may be left in the fermentation crock for another 3 weeks before it is distributed into mason jars.

Use only clean utensils when removing sauerkraut from the pot. Wooden utensils are preferable, as the beneficial bacteria should not come into contact with metal (except for stainless steel).

Sauerkraut Brine

If you're in stage 1 or 2 of the intro diet and wish to make a lot of brine so you can start working on increasing your intake of probiotics (see box, page 28), reduce the cabbage by half and fill the fermentation crock only half-full, then, after smashing the cabbage, fill the jar up with cold-water brine (2% salt). Proceed with step 6. Sip the brine as a supplement or a refreshing drink, or add it to soup (at a maximum temperature of 109°F/43°C).

Store the cabbage, still covered in brine, in the fridge for when you're ready to start eating sauerkraut, or serve it to someone who likes it.

Sauerkraut in a Mason Jar

**Makes about
4 cups (1 L)**

You can multiply this recipe as desired. No matter what amount of cabbage you are fermenting, the ratio of salt per pound or kilogram cabbage should be 2%. Jars should be filled up to the neck, and the cabbage kept below the surface of the brine.

Tips

Be exact when adding salt. Too little may result in slimy cabbage, too much may stop the fermentation. To calculate the quantity of salt you need, weigh the trimmed cabbage in ounces or grams and multiply the weight by 0.02; the resulting number is the weight of salt in ounces or grams you should use.

Use only clean utensils when removing sauerkraut from the pot. Wooden utensils are preferable, as the beneficial bacteria should not come into contact with metal (except for stainless steel).

For information about using sauerkraut brine as a source of probiotics, see the box on page 28.

- *Mandoline*
- *1-quart (1 L) mason jar with airlock lid*
- *Tamper*
- *Black cloth with clothespins*

2 lbs 3 oz	cabbage	1 kg
0.7 oz	pure sea salt or Himalayan salt (approx.)	20 g
	Boiling water	
	Cold-water brine (2% salt), if needed	

1. Rinse outer leaves of cabbage thoroughly to remove all dirt. Remove stem and weigh the remaining cabbage to determine the exact amount of salt needed (see tip).

2. Using a mandoline, cut cabbage into very thin strips. Cut the last bits into thin strips with a sharp knife.

3. Place cabbage strips in a clean, sterilized tall container, such as an old-fashioned pickle jar, and sprinkle with the measured salt. Mix well so the cabbage will macerate.

4. Wash and sterilize the mason jar, all parts of the lid and the tamper with boiling water.

5. Using the tamper, smash cabbage as much as possible in the pickle jar so it is packed down tightly and is macerating.

6. Pack cabbage into the jar, making sure it is covered with brine. If any cabbage is above the brine, add enough cold-water brine to cover.

7. Seal jar with lid and airlock according to the manufacturer's instructions. Wrap jar with a black cloth fastened with clothespins so that only the airlock is sticking out.

8. Store at about 68°F (20°C) for 8 to 10 days, then move it to a cooler place, preferably at 59°F (15°C), for 11 to 13 days (3 weeks total). Continue fermenting for another 3 weeks (6 weeks total). (You can also place the jar in the refrigerator after the first 8 to 10 days, but then it requires fermentation for 11 weeks total.)

9. Consume sauerkraut or store it in a cool, dark place.

Tomato Salsa

Makes about
3 cups (750 mL)

This salsa goes well with a lot of dishes. Serve it whenever you wish to spice up a casserole, as a topping on Carrot and Zucchini Spaghetti (page 182) or as a part of a tapas lunch. Or dip carrot and celery sticks in this probiotic, dairy-free condiment!

Tip

Make sure you use a 3-cup (750 mL) mason jar. A larger jar will not work for this recipe.

- *3-cup (750 mL) mason jar with airlock lid*
- *Tamper*
- *Blender*
- *Black cloth with clothespins*

3	large sun-ripened tomatoes	3
2	cloves garlic, minced	2
1	onion (about 6 oz/175 g), chopped	1
1	fresh hot chile pepper, seeded and chopped	1
1/4 cup	fresh cilantro, chopped	60 mL
1/2 tsp	sea salt	2 mL

Liquid

1	large sun-ripened tomato	1
1	fresh hot chile pepper	1
1	clove garlic	1
2 1/2 tbsp	freshly squeezed lime juice	37 mL

1. Wash and sterilize the mason jar, all parts of the lid and the tamper with boiling water. Let cool while you prepare the salsa.

2. Finely dice tomatoes and transfer them to a large bowl along with their juices. Stir in garlic, onion, chile and cilantro. Sprinkle with salt.

3. *Liquid:* In blender, process tomato, chile, garlic and lime juice. Add liquid to tomato mixture and mix well.

4. Transfer salsa to the jar, filling it to the "shoulders," and, using the tamper, press it down so that the liquid rises to cover the vegetables.

5. Seal jar with lid and airlock according to manufacturer's instructions. Wrap jar with a black cloth fastened with clothespins so that only the airlock is sticking out. Let ferment at room temperature for 48 hours.

6. Consume salsa or store in the refrigerator unopened for up to 3 months or for up to 1 week once opened.

Kimchi

Makes about
3 cups (750 mL)

Kimchi has its origins in the Korean kitchen and may be prepared in a variety of ways, so long as it contains ginger, garlic, onion and chiles. Kimchi tastes great as is or served with Sour Cream (page 92).

Tips

Make sure you use a 3-cup (750 mL) mason jar. A larger jar will not work for this recipe.

Kimchi is typically prepared with Chinese cabbage and radishes, but organic versions of these can be hard to find. To avoid toxins, purchase organic romaine lettuce and carrots, or substitute any other lettuce or cabbage (cabbage must be cut more finely than lettuce) and GAPS-friendly root vegetables.

- *Disposable gloves*
- *3-cup (750 mL) mason jar with airlock lid*
- *Tamper*
- *Black cloth with clothespins*

8 cups	water	2 L
¹⁄₂ cup	salt	125 mL
2	heads romaine lettuce	2
6	carrots (about 10 oz/300 g total)	6
¹⁄₄ cup	grated gingerroot (about 3¹⁄₂ oz/100 g)	60 mL
8	cloves garlic, minced	8
4	fresh hot chile peppers, minced	4
1	large onion, minced	1
	Cold-water brine (3% to 5% salt), if needed	

1. In a large dish, dissolve salt in water.

2. Cut lettuce heads in half lengthwise, remove cores and cut each half lengthwise into thirds. Rinse and cut crosswise into strips about ³⁄₄ inch (2 cm) wide. Place strips in the salt water.

3. Cut carrots into julienne strips, like matchsticks, and add to salt water. Let stand for at least 1¹⁄₂ hours.

4. Drain salt water, rinse vegetables once and let them drain for 5 minutes. They should still taste faintly of salt.

5. Wearing disposable gloves, add ginger, garlic, chiles and onion to the salted vegetables and mix thoroughly.

6. Wash and sterilize the mason jar, all parts of the lid and the tamper with boiling water. Let cool.

Tips

If you are uncertain about the strength of the chile peppers, taste them first and adjust the amount to your taste.

You can substitute 3 tbsp (45 mL) Korean chili powder for the fresh chile peppers.

7. Stuff kimchi into the jar. Using the tamper, press kimchi down so it is covered with brine. The jar should be filled to the "shoulders" and none of the vegetables should be above the brine. If any kimchi is above the brine, add enough cold-water brine to cover.

8. Seal jar with lid and airlock according to manufacturer's instructions. Wrap jar with a black cloth fastened with clothespins so that only the airlock is sticking out. Store at 68°F (20°C) for about 1 week, then move to a cooler place (about 60°F/15°C) and continue fermenting for 3 weeks total or until no air bubbles rise when the jar is slightly tilted.

9. Store kimchi for 3 weeks at a cool temperature (41 to 68°F/5 to 20°C) and it's ready to enjoy. Once opened, store kimchi in the refrigerator for up to 3 months.

Fermenting Milk and Cream

As with fermented vegetables, fermented milk products have been produced all over the world for centuries. They were traditionally made from raw milk, which means it had not been pasteurized (heat-treated) like the milk we buy today. Raw milk contains a multitude of beneficial microbes that are ruined during the pasteurization process. The good news is that you can revive pasteurized milk by fermenting it.

Yogurt, Sour Cream and Kefir in 24 Hours

To prepare dairy products that you can enjoy on the GAPS diet, the recipes in this section will teach you to make:

- yogurt from cow's milk
- sour cream from heavy or whipping (35%) cream
- kefir from cow's milk (or other types of milk, such as goat's milk) or coconut milk

The milk you use should be unhomogenized, full-fat, and organic or biodynamic. Raw milk is ideal, if you are able to obtain it from a milk producer you trust (see box, page 91), and it is also easier to work with than pasteurized milk.

For use on the GAPS diet, all sour milk products should ferment for at least 24 hours, the time required for the milk sugar, lactose, to break down. Store-bought sour milk products have undergone a significantly shorter fermentation process (about 5 to 6 hours).

Whey and Fresh Cheese

The watery part of fermented milk is called whey. In the GAPS diet, homemade whey is highly prized as an important medicinal product, as it contains more types of probiotics than can be extracted into a supplement pill. When you want pure whey, drain yogurt or kefir. Sour cream can also be drained, but it doesn't yield as much whey. Add whey to hot soup (at a maximum temperature of 109°F/43°C), juice and smoothies.

When yogurt, kefir or sour cream has been drained of whey, a white, creamy substance remains that you can use as fresh cheese, cottage cheese or soft-curd cheese if you are able to tolerate a minimal amount of lactose.

About Raw Milk

If raw milk contains beneficial substances, why did we start pasteurizing it in the first place? With intensive agriculture and large herds came adverse consequences to the health of dairy cows, which resulted in more harmful microbes making their way into the cows' milk. Commercial pasteurization was introduced in the late 1800s as a way to both improve the safety of milk and prolong its shelf life.

The trouble is that it's not just harmful microbes that die during the pasteurization process; the beneficial microbes die too, leaving milk that is bereft of the probiotic benefits conveyed by raw milk. Recently, raw milk has been making a comeback, and it is recommended on the GAPS diet — if you can find good-quality milk from a local farmer you trust and who has high standards of hygiene.

Publisher's note: Raw milk is illegal to sell, trade or barter in some U.S. states and in Canada. Even in states where you can legally purchase raw milk, there may be restrictions on sales. If you decide to consume raw milk, please be aware that there are food safety concerns associated with it, which must be balanced against any potential benefits.

Equipment

When making yogurt and sour cream, you will need a food thermometer and a reliable kitchen timer. Use the timer to remind you to keep checking while your milk or cream heats up and subsequently cools down. Note how long each step takes and write it down so that in the future you can just set the timer and not have to constantly check the temperature.

If your oven can be set to between 100°F and 109°F (38°C and 43°C), you can use it to keep the sour milk or cream appropriately lukewarm while it is fermenting. If you need to use the oven for something else during the 24-hour fermentation period, you can remove the pot from the oven and wrap it in a blanket in the meantime, then return the pot to the oven when it's back to the correct temperature. The advantage of using an oven is that you can make larger amounts at a time. But if this doesn't work for you, you might want to purchase a yogurt maker. Alternatively, some people use a slow cooker or a large dehydrator with a thermostat.

Practice good hygiene when fermenting and when eating fermented products.

Fermenting Hygiene

Practice good hygiene when fermenting and when eating fermented products. If using a yogurt maker, wash and sterilize the container before pouring in the milk or cream — every time. Use only clean spoons to remove yogurt or sour cream from its container, and return it immediately to the refrigerator after taking what you need.

Yogurt or Sour Cream

Makes 4 cups (1 L)

Making your own yogurt and sour cream is crucial on the GAPS diet, as 24-hour fermentation makes them almost lactose-free. They contain valuable probiotics and are nourishing when made from good-quality full-fat milk or cream. They're great for breakfast with fresh fruit, nuts, shredded coconut or honey, in or with desserts and baked goods, in soups or as a base for various condiments.

Tips

For the fermentation starter, you can use a store-bought culture, 2 to 3 tbsp (30 to 45 mL) of leftover fermented yogurt or sour cream from the last batch, or a dry fermentation starter (which can be purchased online).

Take advantage of whey's medicinal benefits by adding it to stock, bone broth, soup, fresh juice and smoothies. Do not add probiotics to food that is above 109°F (43°C) or the beneficial bacteria will die.

Consume whey cautiously at the start of the diet. Read "How to Increase Your Intake of Probiotics," page 28.

For Yogurt

| 4 cups | full-fat milk | 1 L |
| | Fermentation starter (see tip) | |

For Sour Cream

| 4 cups | heavy or whipping (35%) cream | 1 L |
| | Fermentation starter (see tip) | |

1. In a pot, heat milk or cream to 181°F (83°C) over medium heat. Remove from heat and let cool to between 109°F and 114°F (43°C and 46°C).

2. Whisk fermentation starter into milk or cream. If using a dry starter, follow the instructions on the package. Cover pot with a lid and place in a 100°F to 109°F (38°C to 43°C) oven. Or pour milk or cream into the container(s) of a yogurt maker and turn it on. Incubate for 24 hours.

3. Let cool to room temperature, then refrigerate until chilled. Store in an airtight container in the refrigerator for up to 12 days.

Variation

Yogurt and Sour Cream from Raw Milk: Heat milk to 109°F (43°C), then continue with step 2. (See box, page 91, for information on raw milk.)

To Make Whey

Pour yogurt (or sour cream) into a colander lined with cheesecloth and let the whey drain off for 24 hours in a cool place. Discard the milk solids or, if you can tolerate a small amount of lactose, use them as fresh cheese, cottage cheese or soft-curd cheese.

Coconut Kefir

**Makes about
2 cups (500 mL)**

*Probiotics are worth their
weight in gold for anyone
following the GAPS diet,
so why not turn coconut
milk into a probiotic food
too? Use this rather thick
coconut kefir to make
ice cream (page 231) or in
cold sauces with herbs and
spices, such as Horseradish
Cream (page 184).*

Tips

In place of the homemade
coconut milk, you can use
a 14-oz (400 mL) can of
organic coconut milk with
no additives.

Kefir remains alive even
when stored, so the flavor
may become more sour
over time.

- *Coffee filters and elastic bands*
- *Mesh strainer (plastic or stainless steel)*

1½ tsp	milk kefir grains	7 mL
2 cups	Coconut Milk (page 76)	500 mL

1. Place kefir grains in the bottom of a clean glass.

2. Whisk coconut milk to keep it from separating and pour over grains. Cover the glass with a coffee filter and secure with an elastic band.

3. Let ferment for 24 hours, away from direct sunlight. Kefir prefers a temperature around 68°F (20°C). Higher temperatures speed up the fermentation process; cooler temperatures slow it down. To determine whether it is fermented enough, taste it. It should have a tangy flavor mixed with the taste of coconut.

4. Set strainer over a measuring cup or bowl. Pour kefir through strainer to catch the grains. Place the unrinsed grains back in a glass that you have used for milk kefir, then start a batch of milk kefir by pouring in cow's milk and covering the glass with a coffee filter secured with an elastic band.

5. Pour the strained coconut kefir into a clean container or bottle, cover with a coffee filter and secure with an elastic band. Store in the refrigerator for up to 1 week.

Kefir

Makes 2 cups (500 mL)

Kefir is a great snack that you can drink. It perks you up, it is satisfying, and it contains probiotics. Kefir is based on milk kefir grains that resemble rice pudding (more or less). The grains contain many different types of bacteria and yeasts, and are sustained by lactose. Combining milk and kefir grains creates a tangy buttermilk flavor and a thick, milky consistency. Thanks to the fermentation, kefir keeps longer, has a fuller taste and agrees with the human gut better than unfermented pasteurized milk.

Tips

Dried kefir fermentation starter may be purchased online.

Even if you are not yet able to tolerate milk kefir, it is still worth making it just for the whey, which is a potent probiotic. But be careful when consuming kefir whey at the start of the diet. It is powerful stuff! Read "How to Increase Your Intake of Probiotics," page 28.

- *1-pint (500 mL) mason jar*
- *Coffee filters and elastic bands*
- *Mesh strainer (plastic or stainless steel)*

1½ tsp	milk kefir grains or dried kefir fermentation starter	7 mL
2 cups	full-fat milk	500 mL

1. Place kefir grains in the bottom of the mason jar. If using a starter, follow the instructions on the package. Pour milk on top. Cover jar with a coffee filter and secure with an elastic band.

2. Let ferment for 24 hours, away from direct sunlight. Kefir prefers a temperature around 68°F (20°C). Higher temperatures speed up the fermentation process; cooler temperatures slow it down. To determine whether it is fermented enough, taste it. It should have a tangy flavor similar to buttermilk.

3. Set strainer over a measuring cup or bowl. Pour kefir through strainer to catch the grains. To start a second batch, place the unrinsed grains back in the unrinsed jar, pour in more fresh milk and cover with a coffee filter secured with an elastic band.

4. Pour the strained kefir into a clean container or bottle, cover with a small piece of coffee filter and secure with an elastic band. Store in the refrigerator for up to 3 weeks. It may separate, but just give it a good shake and it's ready to drink.

To Make Kefir Whey

Pour kefir into a strainer lined with a clean, tightly woven, lint-free tea towel and let the whey drain off for 24 hours in a cool place. Discard the milk solids or, if you can tolerate a small amount of lactose, use them as fresh cheese, cottage cheese or soft-curd cheese.

Tips

Add kefir whey to your daily stock or bone broth, fresh juice, a smoothie or Vallentino's Favorite Drink (page 206). It can also be used for baking bread when you are transitioning out of the GAPS diet.

Kefir remains alive even when stored, so the flavor may become more sour over time.

More Kefir-Making Tips

- Become a member of a Facebook group for people who ferment and make kefir, where you can contact people who want to share their excess kefir grains. The grains multiply, so one day you, too, will be able to give some away. You will, in fact, have to get rid of some so that you don't end up with too many grains in proportion to the milk, which will cause the kefir to separate.

- You can purchase dried kefir grains, but they cannot be reused as many times as the fresh grains.

- If you want to take a break from kefir, you can store the grains with milk, covered, in the refrigerator. They will keep for at least 3 months. Once a week, pour the milk and grains into a clean container and rinse the jar, then return the grain mixture to the rinsed jar. There's no need to wash the jar more often than that, and indeed the kefir won't turn out as well if you do.

- Milk kefir grains can be used in coconut and almond milk, though the resulting kefir will not be 100% dairy-free. But it is important to feed them some cow's milk at regular intervals since they live off lactose!

- Store-bought kefir likely no longer contains live probiotics. Even if it does, it will probably not be as many as in homemade, depending on how it is treated during the production process. So, if you purchase store-bought kefir, don't expect it to be full of probiotics; drink it mainly for its taste and consistency, plus some nourishment, depending on the quality of the milk it is made from.

- I never make water kefir because it lives off sugar and, when it comes to kefir, sugar cannot be replaced with honey. Since I'm not certain whether residual sugar may remain in water kefir, I would rather do without it. Furthermore, I don't feel like making two different kinds of kefir; there are plenty of other things to do in the kitchen when you're on the GAPS diet! The flavor and probiotic benefits of Vallentino's Favorite Drink (page 206) easily match those of water kefir.

Soups and Light Meals

About Bone Broth

Just like fermented foods, our ancestors have sworn by bone broth for millennia. By cooking bone broth and using it as the base for so many dishes, we manage to kill four birds with one stone:

1. It adds fantastic flavor to casseroles, soups and sauces.

2. It helps us maintain good health and contributes to preventing diseases.

3. It is a way to use the entire animal so that none of it goes to waste. Even gnawed bones still have a lot of kick to them and can contribute to good bone broth. Heads, chicken feet, pigs' trotters, cartilage, connective tissue, marrow — just about everything that isn't meat (or fur or feathers!) can be used in a bone broth. (Of course, meat can also be used, but that would mean we were making stock rather than bone broth, and we wouldn't be able to cook it as long to extract more and more of the valuable nutrients.)

4. It can be ready whenever you need it to be. As Sally Fallon Morell and Kaayla T. Daniel write in *Nourishing Broth: An Old-Fashioned Remedy for the Modern World*, food that has simmered for a long time was the original fast food. Since there was always a large pot simmering on the stove, you could easily ladle out a portion whenever you were hungry.

Bone broth is so delicious because it embodies the deep, rich flavor known as umami. These days, there are convenience products, such as bouillon cubes, that mimic the flavor of bone broth and can be used to prepare soups and sauces in a matter of minutes. However, these products cannot replace the gold mine of nutrients found in bone broth. Bone broth that is simmered for 12 to 72 hours contains building blocks for the cells throughout our body, helping us heal and stay healthy.

Stock vs. Bone Broth

Stock is made with meat and some bone, and is simmered for just 1½ to 2 hours so that the meat does not get overcooked and tough. Bone broth, which is made with only a small amount of meat (if any), is simmered for much longer — from 12 to 72 hours — to extract as many nutrients as possible from the bones. From a medicinal point of view, stock has a much milder effect on vulnerable gut tissue. For that reason, you should consume stock, not bone broth, while on the intro diet.

Bone Broth

Makes about 24 cups (6 L)

Drink bone broth daily while on the GAPS diet. Make as large a batch as possible at a time and freeze it in smaller portions. While you're reheating it, add water as needed if you have reduced it, along with salt to taste and maybe a little minced garlic.

Tips

For more deeply flavored broth, place fresh bones in a roasting pan and brown in a 400°F (200°C) oven for 1 hour, turning occasionally. (This step isn't necessary for leftover cooked bones.)

Bone broth is also good as a base for soups, stews or gravies, or mixed into minced meat.

Bone broth based solely on beef bones is, as far as taste goes, rather off-putting, as it is very fatty. But it is excellent as a base for a soup!

See more bone broth tips on page 100.

- *12-quart (12 L) stockpot*
- *Blender (optional)*

6½ to 9 lbs	bones (a mixture of poultry, pork, beef, ox, lamb and game, including chicken feet or a pig's trotter)	3 to 4 kg
8 quarts	cold water (approx.)	8 L
2 tbsp	apple cider vinegar	30 mL
	Fresh or frozen leek tops	
	Parsley stalks	
	Celery top	
2	bay leaves	2
Pinch	salt	Pinch
1 tbsp	whole peppercorns	15 mL

1. Place bones in stockpot, cover with cold water and add vinegar. Bring to a boil over high heat. Reduce heat immediately and simmer for 5 minutes, then skim off and discard any foam that floats to the surface.

2. Add leek tops, parsley, celery top, bay leaves, salt and peppercorns. Cover, reduce heat to low and simmer gently for 12 to 72 hours.

3. Remove from heat and let cool slightly. Strain, leaving as much marrow, cartilage and fat as possible in the broth. If desired, transfer broth to a blender and process to incorporate marrow, cartilage and fat into the broth. (If this sounds unappetizing, just remember that these ingredients have a medicinal effect and are not noticeable once they have been blended in.)

4. To reduce broth, return it to the pot and let it boil, uncovered, over medium-high heat for as long as your patience permits and without letting it totally evaporate! (This step is not necessary, but it will make the broth more concentrated so it won't take up as much room in your freezer.)

5. Refrigerate broth until chilled, then distribute into airtight containers (see tip, page 100). Store in the freezer for up to 1 year.

More Bone Broth Tips

- Save all leftover bones, fat and cartilage from chops, ribs, leg and shoulder roasts, bird carcasses, etc. (including those that have been gnawed), and store in the freezer until you have enough to make broth. Or buy fresh soup bones.

- Pig's trotters and chicken feet are an especially good base for bone broth, as they contain good amounts of gelatin.

- Ask your butcher to crack large joints or bones, or saw them in half, so the marrow may be used.

- Once the bone broth is chilled, you can either pour it into several small containers for freezing, or you can freeze it in a couple of big ones. If you choose big containers, after a couple of days, thaw the frozen broth in the refrigerator for about an hour, then cut the broth into small pieces. Place the pieces in freezer bags, separately so that they don't stick together.

- If the bones contain a lot of gelatin, bone broth turns into a jelly when it is chilled. Cut the cold jelly into squares and freeze them. This jelly also contains many beneficial nutrients and is delicious on pâtés or with other cold meat dishes.

Fish Bone Broth

Makes about 16 cups (4 L)

For fish bone broth, only the bones, heads, fins and tails are used, and it must simmer for at least 4 hours. Use nonfatty white fish, such as cod. You can drink fish bone broth as is (adding salt to taste), add a handful of shrimp or fresh herbs, or use it as a base for fish soup.

Tips

Ask in the fish department if you can buy bones, fins, heads or tails. (They might just let you have them for free!)

Buy whole fish and fillet them or have the fish department do it; make a wonderful dish from the flesh and store the bones, fins, heads and tails in the freezer until you have collected enough to make bone broth.

To prevent bitterness in the broth, you'll need to rinse the fish parts so well that not even a speck of blood remains. Round white fish are easier to rinse well than flat fish.

- **8-quart (8 L) stockpot**

5 lbs	nonfatty white fish heads, bones, fins and tails	2.5 kg
5 quarts	cold water (approx.)	5 L
2 tbsp	apple cider vinegar	30 mL
	Parsley or dill stalks	
Pinch	salt	Pinch
1 tbsp	whole peppercorns	15 mL

1. Rinse fish parts thoroughly in cold water. Place fish parts in stockpot, cover with cold water and add vinegar. Bring to a simmer over medium-low heat. Simmer for 2 minutes, then skim off and discard any foam that floats to the surface.

2. Add parsley, salt and peppercorns. Cover, reduce heat to low and simmer gently for 4 to 24 hours.

3. Remove from heat and let cool slightly. Strain stock and discard solids.

4. To reduce broth, return it to the pot and let it boil, uncovered, over medium-high heat for as long as your patience permits and without letting it totally evaporate! (This step is not necessary, but it will make the broth more concentrated so it won't take up as much room in your freezer.)

5. Refrigerate broth until chilled, then distribute into airtight containers (see tip, page 100). Store in the freezer for up to 6 months.

Chicken or Veal Stock

**Makes about
20 cups (5 L)**

*Stock is based on meat
and bones, and about 80%
of the total weight should
consist of meat. Make as
large a batch as possible
at a time and freeze it in
smaller portions. Drink it
often while on the intro
diet, and add it to soups
and stews.*

Tips

Drink lots of stock while on
the intro diet. While you're
reheating it, add water as
needed if you have reduced
it, along with salt to taste and
maybe a little minced garlic.

The chicken carcass or veal
bones, including cartilage,
can be stored in the freezer
and used to make Bone Broth
(page 99) — the bones are
still potent!

- **8-quart (8 L) stockpot**

2 to 4 lb	large chicken or front cut of veal (such as bone-in mid-rib, breast or shoulder)	1 to 2 kg
6 quarts	cold water (approx.)	6 L
2	onions	2
2	carrots	2
	Parsley stalks or 1 celery top	
1	bay leaf	1
Pinch	salt	Pinch
1 tbsp	whole peppercorns	15 mL

1. Place chicken in stockpot and cover with cold water. Bring to a boil over high heat. Reduce heat immediately and simmer for 3 to 5 minutes, then skim off and discard any foam that floats to the surface.

2. Add onions, carrots, parsley, bay leaf, salt and peppercorns. Cover, reduce heat to low and simmer gently for $1\frac{1}{2}$ to 2 hours or until stock is flavorful.

3. Remove chicken and remove all meat, skin and fat from carcass or bones. (Eat the meat, save it for future meals or freeze it.)

4. Strain stock and discard solids. (Remove onions and carrots to consume.)

5. If desired, reduce stock slightly by returning it to the pot and letting it simmer over medium heat until reduced as desired.

6. Distribute cooled stock into airtight containers (see tip, page 100) and store in the refrigerator for up to 6 days or in the freezer for up to 1 year.

Fish Stock

Makes about
20 cups (5 L)

Both flesh and bones are used to make fish stock; as a GAPS stock, it must simmer for 1½ hours. Drink it as is, or use it as a base for fish soup. This recipe uses cod, but you can replace it with any other nonfatty white fish.

Tips

For a more intense taste and smaller quantity, you can boil the stock to reduce it slightly after straining.

From a medicinal viewpoint, stock is milder than bone broth and is therefore recommended for the intro diet.

- *8-quart (8 L) stockpot*
- *Blender (optional)*

1	large cod head with a small amount of meat from the back of the neck attached (about 4 lbs/2 kg)	1
1	carrot	1
1	onion	1
1½ tbsp	whole peppercorns	22 mL
6 quarts	cold water (approx.)	6 L
	Salt and freshly ground black pepper	

1. Rinse cod head thoroughly in cold water. In stockpot, combine cod head, carrot, onion and peppercorns. Cover with cold water. Bring to a simmer over medium-low heat. Simmer for 5 minutes, then skim off and discard any foam that floats to the surface. Cover, reduce heat to low and simmer for 1½ hours.

2. Remove cod's head to a plate and let cool. Reserve carrot and onion to eat or use as thickener.

3. Strain stock and discard remaining solids. Scoop out flesh from cod's head to use in a separate cod dish, in the stock or in a fish soup.

4. If desired, to thicken the stock, process carrot, onion and a spoonful of stock in blender, then return to the stock.

5. Season stock with salt and pepper to taste.

Stock with Poached Egg

Makes 1 serving

A poached egg has a consistency between soft-cooked and hard-cooked. Who would have thought that such a simple recipe — a bowl of stock with a poached egg — could be so soothing and delicious?

Tips

If you have a larger appetite, you can use up to 1$\frac{2}{3}$ cups (400 mL) stock in this recipe.

To enhance this recipe, you can add chopped fresh parsley and/or well-cooked vegetables.

¾ cup	Chicken or Veal Stock (page 102) or Fish Stock (page 103)	175 mL
Pinch	salt	Pinch
	Freshly ground black pepper	
1	large egg	1
1	clove garlic, crushed	1

1. In a small saucepan, bring stock to a simmer over medium-low heat. Taste and if stock is too concentrated, dilute with some water. Season with salt and with pepper to taste.

2. Carefully crack egg into stock and simmer for 2 minutes or until cooked as desired. Add garlic and cook for a few seconds right before serving.

Variation

Once you are on the full GAPS diet, use Bone Broth (page 99) or Fish Bone Broth (page 101) in place of the stock. At this point, you may also add crisply cooked diced bacon and/or shredded Swiss cheese, if desired.

Fish Stock with Shrimp

Makes 1 serving

When you cook in a GAPS-friendly way, it can sometimes seem like you need to work just as hard in the kitchen as your great-grandmother did. But today we have much more help in the form of kitchen equipment such as blenders and freezers. She would have to boil and peel the shrimp; you can just add ready-to-use shrimp, heat them and eat them.

Tips

If you have a larger appetite, you can use up to 1¼ cups (300 mL) stock in this recipe.

Use small amounts of sauerkraut brine or whey at first — just 1 to 2 tsp (5 to 10 mL) — then gradually increase the amount as your tolerance for probiotics increases.

If you have an immersion blender, you can use it right in the pot in step 2, rather than transferring the stock to a stand blender.

- **Blender (optional)**

¾ cup	Fish Stock (page 103)	175 mL
½	onion, coarsely chopped	½
½	zucchini or yellow summer squash, diced	½
½ cup	frozen peeled and deveined cooked shrimp	125 mL
	Salt and freshly ground black pepper	
	Sauerkraut brine (see page 85) or whey (see page 92)	

1. In a saucepan, combine stock and onion. Bring to a simmer over medium-low heat. Reduce heat to low and simmer for 15 minutes. Add zucchini and simmer for 10 minutes or until vegetables are soft.

2. If desired, for a creamier stock, process in blender, then return to saucepan and return to a simmer.

3. Add shrimp to stock and simmer until heated through. Season to taste with salt and pepper.

4. Remove from heat and let cool to 109°F (43°C). Stir in sauerkraut brine or whey.

Cauliflower Chicken Stock

Makes 1 serving

This combination of a few simple ingredients creates a deep, satisfying flavor that is both healing and a treat for gourmets!

Tips

If you have a larger appetite, you can use up to 1¼ cups (300 mL) stock in this recipe.

Use small amounts of sauerkraut brine or whey at first — just 1 to 2 tsp (5 to 10 mL) — then gradually increase the amount as your tolerance for probiotics increases.

If you have an immersion blender, you can use it right in the pot in step 2, rather than transferring the stock to a stand blender.

• *Blender*

¾ cup	Chicken Stock (page 102)	175 mL
1	carrot, sliced	1
½	onion, coarsely chopped	½
1 cup	cauliflower florets (or more)	250 mL
2	cloves garlic, crushed	2
	Salt and freshly ground black pepper	
	Sauerkraut brine (see page 85) or whey (see page 92)	

1. In a saucepan, combine stock, carrot and onion. Bring to a simmer over medium-low heat. Simmer for 10 minutes. Add cauliflower and simmer for 20 minutes or until vegetables are soft.

2. Transfer stock to blender and process until smooth.

3. Return stock to saucepan, add garlic and season to taste with salt and pepper. Bring to a boil over high heat.

4. Remove from heat and let cool to 109°F (43°C). Stir in sauerkraut brine or whey.

Variation

Once you are in stage 5 of the intro diet, if you tolerate spices, you can add a pinch of freshly grated nutmeg with the garlic.

Mediterranean Stock

Makes 1 serving

Bring this lovely stock with you in an insulated bottle and drink it in sips throughout the day, keeping yourself fortified wherever you are.

Tips

Don't use canned tomatoes in the GAPS diet. Buy crushed tomatoes in glass jars, which are not coated with unwanted chemicals. Freeze any leftovers from the jar for later use.

Use small amounts of sauerkraut brine or whey at first — just 1 to 2 tsp (5 to 10 mL) — then gradually increase the amount as your tolerance for probiotics increases.

If you have an immersion blender, you can use it right in the pot in step 2, rather than transferring the stock to a stand blender.

• **Blender**

¾ cup	Chicken Stock (page 102) or Fish Stock (page 103)	175 mL
½ cup	crushed tomatoes (from a jar)	125 mL
1	small carrot, diced	1
1	slice celery root, diced	1
½	onion, coarsely chopped	½
1	clove garlic, crushed	1
	Salt and freshly ground black pepper	
	Sauerkraut brine (see page 85) or whey (see page 92)	

1. In a saucepan, combine stock, tomatoes, carrot, celery root and onion. Bring to a simmer over medium-low heat. Simmer for 30 minutes (reducing heat to low if using fish stock), until vegetables are soft.

2. Transfer stock to blender and process until smooth.

3. Return stock to saucepan, add garlic and season to taste with salt and pepper. Bring to a boil over high heat.

4. Remove from heat and let cool to 109°F (43°C). Stir in sauerkraut brine or whey.

Fish Soup with Fennel

<table>
<tr><td></td><td>Butter or Clarified Butter (page 68)</td><td></td></tr>
<tr><td>1</td><td>onion, chopped</td><td>1</td></tr>
<tr><td>1</td><td>bulb fennel, finely diced</td><td>1</td></tr>
<tr><td>2</td><td>cloves garlic, minced</td><td>2</td></tr>
<tr><td>4 cups</td><td>Fish Stock (page 103)</td><td>1 L</td></tr>
<tr><td>10 to 14 oz</td><td>cooked fish, cut into small pieces</td><td>300 to 400 g</td></tr>
<tr><td></td><td>Salt and freshly ground black pepper</td><td></td></tr>
<tr><td>1</td><td>clove garlic, crushed (optional)</td><td>1</td></tr>
<tr><td></td><td>Chopped fresh parsley</td><td></td></tr>
</table>

Makes 4 servings

Anise-like flavors, such as dill or fenugreek, match fish and shellfish brilliantly. In this soup, fennel provides an extra-delicate anise taste. As fennel is fairly fibrous, cook it until very soft (unless you are well into the diet and have become a hard-core raw vegetable eater).

Tips

If using raw fish instead of cooked, simmer it in the soup for about 5 minutes or until fish is opaque and flakes easily when tested with a fork.

Serve with soft-cooked eggs.

1. In a medium saucepan over medium-high heat, melt enough butter to make a generous layer. Add onion and fennel; cook, stirring, for about 5 minutes or until tender. Add minced garlic and cook, stirring, for 1 minute.

2. Stir in stock and bring to a boil. Reduce heat to medium-low, cover and simmer for at least 20 minutes or until vegetables are soft.

3. Stir in fish and simmer for 2 to 3 minutes to heat through. Season to taste with salt and pepper. If desired, add crushed garlic and cook for 30 seconds.

4. Serve with a bowl of chopped parsley to sprinkle over the soup.

Shrimp Bisque

Makes 2 servings

Never waste an opportunity to make a luxurious bisque, a creamy soup based on shellfish. This version is made with leftover shrimp shells. Whenever you are lucky enough to get hold of some shrimp, fresh or frozen, save the shells that you peel off and store them in the freezer until you have enough to make bisque. Like magic, waste turns into a real delicacy!

Tips

Use between 2 and 6 tbsp (30 and 90 mL) Clarified Butter in step 1, depending on your preference and how much fat you need in your diet.

All kinds of crustacean shells may be used in place of or in addition to the shrimp shells.

	Clarified Butter (page 68)	
4 to 6 cups	shrimp shells	1 to 1.5 L
1	shallot or small onion, finely chopped	1
1/4 to 1/2 cup	dry white wine	60 to 125 mL
	Water	
1 tbsp	Sour Cream (page 92)	15 mL
	Salt and freshly ground pepper	

1. In a medium saucepan, melt desired amount of clarified butter (see tip) over medium-high heat. Add shrimp shells and cook, stirring, for about 5 minutes or until they turn pink.

2. Reduce heat to medium. Add shallot, wine and just enough water to cover; bring to a simmer. Reduce heat to low, cover and simmer for 20 minutes.

3. Strain bisque, discarding solids, and return broth to pan. Taste and, if necessary, boil to reduce liquid and concentrate flavor. Stir in sour cream and season to taste with salt and pepper.

Beef Vegetable Soup

Makes 10 servings		

This soup is a real classic! It's been nourishing people all over the world for as long as there have been pots and fires.

Tips

After removing the cooked carrots and celery root from the broth, you may chop or slice them and eat them immediately; reserve them for the next day's lunch, sautéed in a bit of butter and garlic; use them in an omelet; or mash them with butter and spices.

If you are on the full GAPS diet, you can serve the soup garnished with plenty of freshly grated horseradish.

Store leftovers in airtight containers in the refrigerator for up to 5 days or in the freezer for up to 1 year.

Broth

2 lbs	boneless beef brisket	1 kg
16 cups	cold water	4 L
4	carrots	4
3	leek tops	3
$\frac{1}{2}$	celery root	$\frac{1}{2}$
10 to 20	parsley stalks	10 to 20
	Small handful of peppercorns	
Pinch	salt	Pinch

Soup

4	carrots, diced	4
$\frac{1}{2}$	celery root, diced	$\frac{1}{2}$
2	leeks (white and light green parts only), thinly sliced into rings	2

1. *Broth:* In a large pot, combine brisket and cold water. Bring to a boil over high heat. Reduce heat immediately and simmer for 2 to 3 minutes, then skim off and discard any foam that floats to the surface.

2. Add carrots, leek tops, celery root, parsley, peppercorns and salt. Reduce heat and let simmer for 2 hours or until beef is tender.

3. Transfer brisket to a cutting board. Remove vegetables from broth; discard leek tops and reserve carrots and celery root, if desired (see tip).

4. *Soup:* Return broth to medium-high heat and bring to a boil. Add diced carrots and celery root; reduce heat and simmer for 12 to 15 minutes or until slightly tender. Add sliced leeks and boil for 10 minutes or until vegetables are soft.

5. Slice brisket and return beef to soup. Reduce heat to medium and cook for 2 minutes.

Cauliflower Soup

Makes 6 to 8 servings

This soup makes a delicious starter or a really nice lunch. Make a large batch and take leftovers with you when you're on the go. It tastes great as is, but may also be topped with a poached egg or sprinkled with grated Parmesan cheese or crisply cooked diced bacon.

Tips

Use between 2 and 6 tbsp (30 and 90 mL) cooking fat in step 4, depending on your preference and how much fat you need in your diet.

If you have an immersion blender, you can use it right in the pot in step 6, rather than transferring the soup to a stand blender.

Variation

Substitute Chicken or Veal Stock (page 102) for the bone broth and enjoy the soup from stage 3 of the intro diet.

- *Blender*

6 cups	water	1.5 L
	Salt	
1	medium to large head cauliflower, quartered	1
	Cooking fat	
1	small onion, finely chopped	1
1	large carrot, diced	1
1	stalk celery, diced	1
3	cloves garlic, minced	3
1 cup	Bone Broth (page 99)	250 mL
	Freshly grated nutmeg	
	Freshly ground black pepper	
	Chopped fresh parsley	

1. In a large pot, bring water to a boil over high heat. Season lightly with salt. Add cauliflower and return to a boil; cover and boil for $1\frac{1}{2}$ minutes.

2. Using a slotted spoon, transfer cauliflower to a strainer, reserving cooking water. Rinse cauliflower with cold water to stop cooking process. Let drain.

3. Cut small florets off a quarter of the blanched cauliflower. Place in a bowl and set aside. Cut the remaining cauliflower, including the stem, into smaller but still coarse pieces.

4. In a large saucepan, heat desired amount of cooking fat (see tip) over medium-high heat. Add onion, carrot and celery; cook, stirring, for about 4 minutes or until onion is translucent. Stir in coarsely chopped cauliflower.

5. Stir in garlic, bone broth and reserved cooking water; bring to a boil. Reduce heat and simmer for about 20 minutes or until vegetables are soft.

6. In batches as necessary, transfer soup to blender and process until smooth.

7. Return soup to the saucepan and add nutmeg, salt and pepper to taste. Add reserved cauliflower florets and bring soup to a boil over medium heat. Boil for 2 to 5 minutes or until florets are cooked as desired.

8. Serve with a bowl of chopped parsley to sprinkle over the soup.

Hokkaido Squash Soup

Makes 4 servings

Both children and adults will love this soup and will be pleading for more whenever you serve it.

Tips

If you have Baked Pumpkin or Squash (page 77) in the freezer, you can make this soup at lightning speed. Use 3 cups (750 mL) in place of the whole squash and reduce the cooking time in step 2 to 10 minutes.

If you have an immersion blender, you can use it right in the pot in step 3, rather than transferring the soup to a stand blender.

• *Blender*

¼ cup	coconut oil	60 mL
1	1½-inch (4 cm) piece gingerroot, grated	1
1 tbsp	curry powder	15 mL
1 tsp	ground turmeric	5 mL
1 tsp	ground or crushed coriander seeds	5 mL
Pinch	freshly grated nutmeg	Pinch
	Salt and freshly ground black pepper	
1	Hokkaido, Red Kuri or other winter squash (about 1 lb/500 g), peeled and chopped	1
3	cloves garlic, minced	3
2 cups	Bone Broth (page 99)	500 mL
1⅔ cups	Coconut Milk (page 76)	400 mL
	Grated zest of ½ lime	
	Juice of 1 lime	
	Chopped fresh cilantro	

1. In a medium saucepan, melt coconut oil over medium-high heat. Add ginger, curry powder, turmeric, coriander, nutmeg, and salt and pepper to taste, stirring into a paste. Add squash and cook, stirring, for 1 to 2 minutes or until coated in spices. Add garlic and cook, stirring, for 20 seconds.

2. Stir in bone broth; bring to a boil. Reduce heat to low, cover and simmer for 20 minutes or until squash is soft.

3. In batches as necessary, transfer soup to blender and process until smooth.

4. Return soup to saucepan and stir in coconut milk, lime zest and lime juice. Bring to a boil over medium heat, stirring often.

5. Serve with a bowl of chopped cilantro to sprinkle over the soup.

Tomato Soup

Makes 4 servings

This soup is good all year round. Once you have made it a couple of times, it is pretty easy to cook, as you don't need to start from scratch. Ease the workload by using bottled crushed tomatoes with no additives. Of course, you can use ripe fresh tomatoes if you prefer, but then you need to blanch and peel them first. Serve soup as is or top with grated cheese, a poached egg or chopped fresh parsley.

Tips

Use between 2 and 4 tbsp (30 and 60 mL) cooking fat in step 1, depending on your preference and how much fat you need in your diet.

Don't use canned tomatoes in the GAPS diet. Buy crushed tomatoes in glass bottles, which are not coated with unwanted chemicals. Freeze any leftovers from the bottle for later use.

If you have an immersion blender, you can use it right in the pot in step 3, rather than transferring the soup to a stand blender.

- **Blender**

	Cooking fat	
1	small onion, diced	1
1	carrot, diced	1
1	slice celery root (or 1 stalk celery), diced	1
2	cloves garlic, minced	2
1¼ cups	bottled crushed tomatoes	300 mL
1 cup	Bone Broth (page 99)	250 mL
¾ cup	water	175 mL
¼ to ½ tsp	dried thyme	1 to 2 mL
	Salt and freshly ground black pepper	
1	small drop tomato vinegar (optional)	1

1. In a medium saucepan, heat desired amount of cooking fat (see tip) over medium-high heat. Add onion, carrot and celery root; cook, stirring, for 4 minutes or until onion is translucent. Add garlic and cook, stirring, for 1 minute.

2. Stir in tomatoes, bone broth and water. Season to taste with thyme, salt and pepper. Bring to a boil. Reduce heat and simmer for 20 minutes or until vegetables are soft.

3. In batches as necessary, transfer soup to blender and process until smooth.

4. Return soup to saucepan and reheat until steaming. Taste and adjusting seasoning with thyme, salt, pepper and tomato vinegar, if using.

Variation

Substitute Chicken or Veal Stock (page 102) for the bone broth and enjoy the soup from stage 3 of the intro diet.

Lunch Wraps

**Makes 2 wraps
per variation**

*When you want to make
something special for your
own or your child's lunch
box, these wraps stuffed
with crisp salad and your
favorite filling are a
real treat.*

Tips

For these flourless pancakes,
it may be helpful to use a
crêpe spreader to spread the
batter evenly in the skillet.
A crêpe spatula (an oblong
palette knife, usually made of
wood) will make it easier to
flip them.

To easily remove the pancake
from the skillet and turn it
over, use a crêpe spatula
to slide the pancake onto a
lid, then invert it back into
the skillet.

Don't forget the crisp greens,
which add a bit of crunchy
texture to the wrap.

- *8-inch (20 cm) skillet*

4	large eggs	4
2 tbsp	Sour Cream (page 92)	30 mL
	Cooking fat	

With Salmon Filling (Intro Diet, Stage 5)

½	avocado, sliced	½
	Green lettuce or baby spinach	
6	slices cucumber, cut into strips	6
4 to 6	slices Gravlax (page 121)	4 to 6
	Freshly ground black pepper	

With Chicken Filling (Full GAPS Diet)

½	avocado, sliced	½
	Green lettuce or baby spinach	
¼	red bell pepper, cut into strips	¼
2	slices cooked chicken	2
1 tsp	curry powder	5 mL
2	slices bacon, cooked	2

With Ham and Cheese Filling (Full GAPS Diet)

½	avocado, sliced	½
	Green lettuce or baby spinach	
¼	red bell pepper, cut into strips	¼
2	slices air-dried ham	2
2	slices Swiss cheese or hard goat or sheep cheese	2
	Dijon mustard	

1. In a small bowl, whisk eggs and sour cream until well blended.

2. In the skillet, heat a generous layer of cooking fat over medium heat. Pour in half the egg mixture; cook for 2 to 3 minutes or until golden brown on the bottom. Remove pancake from skillet (see tip), add more fat to skillet, then invert pancake back into skillet. Cook for about 2 minutes or until pancake is set and light brown.

3. Repeat step 2 with the remaining egg mixture, adding more fat and adjusting heat as necessary between pancakes. Let cool.

Tips

There are many other possibilities for fillings, such as sliced fish cakes, well-done vegetables, falafels, meatballs or any sort of sliced roast meat or poultry.

If you happen to have Gravlax Sauce (page 184), Spicy Soft-Curd Cheese (page 196) or Pesto (page 191), those would go very well with these wraps.

4. Cut off about 20 inches (50 cm) of parchment paper and cut in half lengthwise. Fold each piece sharply twice lengthwise. These strips will help hold the wraps together.

5. To assemble each wrap, imagine that the pancake has been cut in half crosswise and the upper half of the circle has been cut into thirds. The filling should be placed in the top middle section. First place half the avocado in that section, then top with half of the remaining filling ingredients, in the order they are called for.

6. Fold the lower half of the pancake over the top half so that the filling is covered. Then fold both sides across the middle. Wrap a parchment paper strip tightly around the lower part of the wrap and fasten it with tape. Wrap the whole thing in another sheet of parchment paper and fasten with a rubber band to prevent the filling from falling out.

7. Repeat steps 5 and 6 with the remaining pancake and filling.

Additional Variations

Salmon Filling for Stage 3: Omit the green lettuce or baby spinach and the cucumber. Instead, use 10 green beans, boiled in salted water until tender, cooled and patted dry, or 2 cups (500 mL) spinach leaves, steamed for 4 minutes, cooled, patted dry and coarsely chopped.

Chicken Filling for Stage 3: In place of the filling ingredients listed on page 114, use 2 slices of well-done chicken (from making stock, for example), well-cooked sliced onion and salt to taste. To prepare the onion, slice a small onion and sauté it in 2 tbsp (30 mL) poultry fat or Clarified Butter (page 68) for 20 to 30 minutes, until very tender, then let cool. If desired, you can add a few chopped mushrooms during the last 10 minutes of sautéing the onion.

Pizza Omelet

This omelet is one of my daughter's favorite recipes. At 12 years old, she has made it herself plenty of times, following the recipe step by step. It is easiest if you have a crêpe pan and a crêpe spatula. You might need to practice the turning technique a few times before you master it.

Tips

To easily remove the omelet from the skillet and turn it over, use a spatula to slide the omelet onto a lid, then invert it back into the skillet.

There are plenty of possible variations for this omelet. Prepare it with or without herbs, spices or cheese, and/or serve it with fish, vegetables or GAPS-friendly bacon, sausage or ham.

• *Electric mixer*

2	large eggs, separated	2
	Butter, Clarified Butter (page 68) or animal fat	
1	tomato, sliced	1
¼ tsp	dried thyme	1 mL
½ cup	shredded Swiss cheese	125 mL

1. In a small bowl, using the electric mixer, beat egg whites until stiff. Carefully fold in egg yolks.

2. In a skillet, melt plenty of butter over medium heat. Pour in egg mixture. Place tomato slices on top and sprinkle with thyme and cheese. Cook for about 3 minutes or until light brown on the bottom. Remove omelet from skillet (see tip), add more butter to skillet, then invert omelet back into skillet. Cook for about 2 minutes or until omelet is set.

Smiling Eggs with Mustard Mayo

Makes 4 servings

A "smiling egg" is a Danish term for an egg cooked somewhere between soft- and hard-cooked. The yolk still has a bright yellow color, and it is still very soft but not runny. Why do we call it a smiling egg? Perhaps because it makes us smile to eat something that has such a delightful flavor and texture, gives us so much satisfaction and is so easy to digest.

Tip
Nice as a starter or as part of your lunch.

4	large eggs	4
2 tbsp	Mayonnaise (page 187)	30 mL
1 tbsp	Dijon mustard	15 mL
	Chopped fresh parsley	

1. Place eggs in a saucepan and add cold water to cover. Bring to a boil over high heat. Boil for 5 minutes or until the outer edges of the whites and yolks are hard and the center of the yolks are soft. Drain and chill in cold water, then peel eggs and cut in half.

2. In a small bowl, stir together mayonnaise and mustard.

3. Dollop mayonnaise mixture on each egg half and sprinkle with parsley.

Spinach Pancakes

Serve these delicious pancakes as an accompaniment to soups and salads, or stuff them with lamb (page 168) for a satisfying dinner. You may need to practice cooking flourless pancakes for a while before they turn out perfect, but you'll soon get the hang of it!

Tips

If you have fresh spinach on hand, do use it! You will need to rinse it well and blanch it for 1 minute, then drain and squeeze it dry before chopping it.

For these flourless pancakes, it may be helpful to use a crêpe spreader to spread the batter evenly in the skillet. A crêpe spatula (an oblong palette knife, usually made of wood) will make it easier to flip them.

To easily remove the pancake from the skillet and turn it over, use a crêpe spatula to slide the pancake onto a lid, then invert it back into the skillet.

6	large eggs	6
2 tbsp	Sour Cream (page 92) or almond butter	30 mL
8 oz	thawed frozen spinach, squeezed dry and chopped	250 g
Pinch	salt	Pinch
	Animal fat, butter or Clarified Butter (page 68)	

1. In a bowl, whisk eggs and sour cream until blended. Stir in spinach and salt.

2. In a medium skillet, heat a generous layer of fat over medium heat. Pour in one-quarter of the egg mixture and cook for 3 to 5 minutes or until light brown on the bottom. Remove pancake from skillet (see tip), add more fat to skillet, then invert pancake back into skillet. Cook for about 3 minutes or until pancake is set and light brown.

3. Repeat step 2 three times with the remaining egg mixture, adding more fat and adjusting heat as necessary between pancakes.

Zucchini Pancakes

Makes 2 pancakes

These pancakes are nice for breakfast, lunch or supper, or you can enjoy them as a snack if you need something between meals.

Tips

Substitute ½ cup (125 mL) Baked Pumpkin or Squash (page 77) for the zucchini and skip step 1.

For these flourless pancakes, it may be helpful to use a crêpe spreader to spread the batter evenly in the skillet. A crêpe spatula (an oblong palette knife, usually made of wood) will make it easier to flip them.

• **Blender**

1	2½-inch (6 cm) piece zucchini or yellow summer squash, peeled	1
2	large eggs	2
1 tsp	peanut or almond butter (optional)	5 mL
Pinch	salt	Pinch
	Animal fat, coconut oil, butter or Clarified Butter (page 68)	

1. In blender, process zucchini until finely chopped.

2. In a bowl, whisk eggs with peanut butter and salt until well blended. Stir in zucchini.

3. In a medium skillet, heat a generous layer of fat over medium heat. Pour in half the egg mixture and cook for 3 to 5 minutes or until golden brown on the bottom. Remove pancake from skillet (see tip, page 118), add more fat to skillet, then invert pancake back into skillet. Cook for about 3 minutes or until pancake is set and light brown.

4. Repeat step 3 with the remaining egg mixture, adding more fat and adjusting heat as necessary between pancakes.

Pumpkin Blinis

Makes 6 blinis

These pancakes are a satisfying accompaniment to soups and salads, or you can use them to make burgers (see box).

Tip
In place of the sour cream, you can substitute 1 tbsp (15 mL) additional beaten egg.

- **Nut grinder (see box, page 75)**

2½ oz	dried soaked hazelnuts (see page 74)	75 g
¾ cup	Baked Pumpkin or Squash (page 77), mashed	175 mL
2	large eggs, beaten	2
1 tbsp	Sour Cream (page 92)	15 mL
1 tsp	curry powder	5 mL
Pinch	salt	Pinch
	Freshly ground black pepper	
	Animal fat, butter or Clarified Butter (page 68)	

1. In nut grinder, grind hazelnuts into fine flour.

2. In a medium bowl, whisk together hazelnut flour, pumpkin, eggs, sour cream, curry powder, salt and plenty of pepper.

3. In a medium skillet, melt fat over medium heat. Working in batches, pour in about one-sixth of the batter per blini, spacing them apart and spreading to 4 inches (10 cm) in diameter. They should be rather thick. Cook for about 5 minutes per side or until golden. Serve warm or, if making burgers, transfer to a wire rack and let cool.

4. Repeat step 3 with the remaining batter, adding more fat and adjusting heat as necessary between blinis.

Burgers on Pumpkin Blinis
Spread a homemade cold sauce, such as Ketchup (page 190), Aïoli (page 188) or Pesto (page 191), on a blini. Place a small, flat hamburger on top, garnish with fresh lettuce, cucumber, slices of tomato and soft or raw onions, then place another pumpkin blini on top.

Gravlax

Makes 10 to
14 servings

*Swedish fishermen used to
bury lightly salted, cleaned
fish wrapped in birch bark
in holes dug in the ground.
This almost salt-free way to
preserve fish was a smart
idea, as salt was scarce.
Even today, we can hardly
improve on that method,
though we wrap the fish
in plastic wrap instead of
bark and use a refrigerator
instead of burying it!
This no-heat preparation
ensures that the fish's
nutrients and oil content
are preserved.*

Tips

Mackerel and Greenland
halibut (Greenland turbot)
are also good candidates for
making gravlax.

Don't use fresh fish; it must
have been frozen for at least
12 days to kill any unwanted
microbes. Let thaw in the
refrigerator for about 6 hours
before preparing the recipe.

When you are on the full
GAPS diet, Gravlax Sauce
(page 184) is wonderful with
slices of gravlax.

Be very careful to observe
good hygiene during this
process and whenever
handling fish.

- *Fillet knife*

1	frozen salmon fillet (1 to $1\frac{1}{2}$ lbs/ 500 to 750 g), thawed and patted dry	1
1	bunch fresh dill (or 2 tbsp/30 mL dried dillweed)	1
1 tbsp	sea salt	15 mL
1 tbsp	crushed green peppercorns (optional)	15 mL
1 tbsp	raw honey	15 mL

1. Cut salmon in half lengthwise or crosswise, depending on the shape of your dish (use a dish that will fit in your refrigerator). Place one half in dish, skin side down.

2. If using fresh dill, soak dill for a couple of minutes, then rinse well. Shake off excess water and rinse again. Pat dill dry, then mince.

3. In a medium bowl, stir dill, salt, pepper (if using) and honey into a paste.

4. Carefully rub paste all over flesh side of salmon in dish. Place the other salmon half on top, skin side up. Cover dish with plastic wrap and refrigerate for 48 hours.

To Carve

5. Place one salmon half on a cutting board, skin side down. Scrape off the dill paste from the portion of fish you want to use. Using the fillet knife, carve off thin slices of salmon, removing them from the skin but leaving skin attached to the remaining fish.

6. Return remaining salmon to dish, covering with skin. Cover dish and refrigerate for up to 5 days.

Lumpfish Roe with Avocado

Makes 2 to 4 servings

Buy lumpfish roe in season, when it is cheapest, and stretch the season with the help of your freezer. At 0°F (–18°C), the roe will keep fine for a couple of months.

Tips

If cleaned roe is not available, you can clean it yourself: pour it into plenty of cold water and whisk it with an egg beater, then remove membranes.

Use between 2 and 4 tbsp (30 and 60 mL) cooking fat in step 2, depending on your preference and how much fat you need in your diet.

Serve roe immediately, as it has a short shelf life at room temperature.

When you are able to tolerate raw onion, you can skip the cooking in step 2.

	Clarified Butter (page 68)	
1	small red onion, very finely chopped	1
7 oz	cleaned lumpfish roe	200 g
2 to 4	large eggs (1 per person)	2 to 4
2 tbsp	freshly squeezed lemon juice, divided	30 mL
	Salt and freshly ground black pepper	
1 to 2	avocados (1/2 per person)	1 to 2

1. In a small saucepan, melt desired amount of clarified butter (see tip) over low heat. Add onion and cook, stirring occasionally, for 20 minutes, until very soft. Transfer to a medium bowl and let cool.

2. Place roe in a sieve, rinse in cold water and let drain.

3. In a medium saucepan, bring about 2 inches (5 cm) of water to a boil over high heat. Reduce heat to low, add eggs in the shell and simmer gently for 6 minutes or to desired doneness. Let cool and peel.

4. To onion, add roe, 1 tbsp (15 mL) lemon juice, and salt and pepper to taste. Refrigerate while preparing avocados.

5. Cut avocados in half, then into canoe-shaped wedges. Drizzle with the remaining lemon juice.

6. Serve roe, avocados and eggs on one attractive platter or as individual servings.

Variation

In place of the eggs, serve each portion with 1 tbsp (15 mL) Sour Cream (page 92).

GAPS Sushi

Makes about 36 pieces		

Serve these delicious pieces of sushi with Horseradish Cream (page 184), which is a pretty good substitute for wasabi.

Tips

As an alternative to the celery strips, you can use toothpicks to spear the sushi rolls.

Use gravlax made from either salmon or Greenland halibut (Greenland turbot) for this recipe.

2	stalks celery, cut into long, very thin strips (see tip)	2
	Cooking fat	
2	large eggs, whisked	2
1	cucumber	1
1	carrot	1
2	avocados	2
24	2- by 1-inch (5 by 2.5 cm) slices Gravlax (page 121)	24
12	fresh or thawed frozen shrimp, peeled, deveined and patted dry	12
36	green peas, patted dry	36

1. In a large pot of boiling salted water, blanch celery for 30 seconds. Drain, let cool and pat dry. These strips are used to tie together the sushi pieces.

2. In a small skillet, heat a thin layer of cooking fat over medium heat. Pour in eggs and cook, without stirring, for about 5 minutes or until omelet is set.

3. Transfer omelet to a cutting board and let cool, then cut into small rectangular pieces, about 2 by 1 inches (5 by 2.5 cm).

4. Using a vegetable peeler, cut 1-inch (2.5 cm) wide strips of cucumber and carrot (the carrot strips should be ultra-thin). Cut the strips crosswise into 2-inch (5 cm) long pieces. (Alternatively, the cucumber strips may be kept long and wrapped around sushi pieces.)

5. Cut avocados into small pieces.

6. For each piece of sushi, stack 1 slice of gravlax or 1 shrimp, 1 piece of omelet, 1 carrot strip, 1 cucumber strip and 1 avocado piece. Tie into a bundle with a cooked celery strip. (Alternatively, wrap cucumber strips around stacks, then tie with celery strips.) Place a pea on top of each bundle.

Jazzed-Up Shrimp

Makes 2 servings

Served with a little sour cream and a green salad, this makes a beautiful appetizer or lunch dish.

Tip

Use between 2 and 4 tbsp (30 and 60 mL) Clarified Butter in step 1, depending on your preference and how much fat you need in your diet.

	Clarified Butter (page 68)	
1	long red chile pepper (medium heat), thinly sliced	1
1	large clove garlic, thinly sliced	1
5 oz	fresh or thawed frozen shrimp, peeled, deveined and patted dry	150 g

1. In a small skillet, melt desired amount of clarified butter (see tip) over low heat. Remove from heat and add chile pepper and garlic. Let stand for 1 hour to infuse flavor.

2. Return skillet to low heat and cook, stirring often, for 5 minutes or until softened. Be careful not to burn garlic.

3. Increase heat to high, add shrimp and cook, stirring, for about 1 minute or until shrimp are pink and opaque. Serve immediately.

Chicken Liver Pâté

Makes 8 servings

You don't need an oven to make this chicken pâté! It should be served cold and is a nice addition to a picnic basket or lunch box. It tastes great with hazelnuts, olives, cucumber salad or sauerkraut.

Tips

You may substitute chicken hearts for some of the chicken livers.

Tomato vinegar can be purchased online. It adds a wonderful umami flavor, but if you don't have it on hand, you can substitute a good-quality no-sugar-added balsamic vinegar.

Store pâté in the refrigerator for up to 5 days or in the freezer for up to 3 months.

- **Blender**
- **Two 1½- to 2-cup (375 to 500 mL) pâté molds**

	Butter, Clarified Butter (page 68) or other animal fat	
1 lb	chicken livers, trimmed	500 g
1 tsp	dried thyme (approx.)	5 mL
	Salt and freshly ground black pepper	
2 tbsp	tomato vinegar (approx.)	30 mL
1	onion, chopped	1
15 oz	mushrooms, diced	450 g

1. In a large skillet, melt 2 tbsp (30 mL) butter over high heat. Add livers and cook for 2 minutes or until browned on one side. Season with thyme, salt and pepper. Turn livers over and cook for 2 minutes or until browned on the other side.

2. Stir in tomato vinegar. Reduce heat to low, cover and simmer for 15 minutes. Transfer livers to blender and set aside.

3. Return skillet to medium-low heat. Add more butter to the pan, if necessary to coat. Add onion and cook, stirring often, for about 10 minutes or until tender.

4. Transfer onion to blender and add 3 tbsp (45 mL) butter or clarified butter. Purée until smooth. Transfer to a large bowl and set aside.

5. In same skillet, melt 2 tbsp (30 mL) butter over medium-high heat. Add mushrooms and season with salt and pepper; cook, stirring often, for about 8 minutes or until liquid is released and mushrooms are lightly browned.

6. Add mushrooms to liver purée and stir well. Taste and adjust seasoning with thyme, salt, pepper and/or tomato vinegar as desired.

7. Spoon liver purée into pâté molds, pressing down lightly, and let cool. Cover and refrigerate until set and chilled, about 2 hours.

Beef or Veal Liver Pâté

Makes 24 servings

Liver is a highly recommended part of the GAPS diet thanks to its high vitamin B$_{12}$ and iron content, which is unmatched by any other food. Some people even make small balls of frozen raw liver, which they swallow daily like pills.

Tips

If you don't have a meat grinder, ask your butcher to grind the liver and lard for you. In step 2, combine them with the ground meat and finely chopped onion in a large bowl.

Tomato vinegar can be purchased online. It adds a wonderful umami flavor, but if you don't have it on hand, you can substitute a good-quality no-sugar-added balsamic vinegar.

- *Preheat oven to 340°F (170°C), with rack set in second-lowest position*
- *Meat grinder (see tip)*
- *Fine-mesh sieve*
- *6 small (1½-cup/375 mL) or 2 large (6- to 8-cup/1.5 to 2 L) ovenproof pâté molds*

2 tbsp	butter or other animal fat	30 mL
8 oz	mushrooms, chopped	250 g
2 lbs	beef or veal liver, trimmed	1 kg
14 oz	lard	400 g
1 lb	ground pork, veal or beef (not lean)	500 g
1	large onion, coarsely chopped	1
5 to 10	oil-packed anchovies, drained	5 to 10
3	cloves garlic, minced (approx.)	3
3	large eggs, beaten	3
½ cup	Sour Cream (page 92)	125 mL
1 tbsp	tomato vinegar (approx.)	15 mL
½ tsp	dried thyme (approx.)	2 mL
	Freshly ground black pepper	
6 to 12	thin slices bacon	6 to 12
	Salt	

1. In a large skillet, melt butter over medium-high heat. Add mushrooms and cook, stirring, for about 8 minutes or until lightly browned. Let cool.

2. Run liver and lard alternately with ground meat and onion through meat grinder into a large bowl.

3. Press anchovies through a fine-mesh sieve into the liver mixture, then stir in along with garlic. Add eggs, sour cream, tomato vinegar and thyme, stirring well. Stir in mushrooms, including any liquid. Season with pepper.

4. Form a small amount of the liver mixture into a ball. In skillet, fry meatball over medium heat until no longer pink inside. Taste meatball and adjust seasoning of remaining liver mixture with garlic, thyme, pepper, salt and/or tomato vinegar as desired.

Tips

This pâté is well suited for freezing, so you can stockpile it for future use. Wrap cooled pâtés well and freeze for up to 3 months. Let thaw in the refrigerator overnight.

You can also freeze the pâtés before baking. That way, when you want freshly baked, warm pâté for a special occasion, you can thaw it overnight in the refrigerator, then bake it just before your guests arrive.

5. Pack liver mixture into pâté molds, dividing equally, and arrange bacon on top.

6. Bake in preheated oven for 75 minutes or until a meat thermometer inserted in the center of a mold registers at least 160°F (71°C). Let pâtés cool in molds until lukewarm, or let cool completely and chill to serve cold.

Variations

If you omit the bacon, this recipe can be enjoyed as of stage 3 of the intro diet.

If you cannot tolerate egg whites, replace each whole egg with 1 egg yolk and 3 tbsp (45 mL) Bone Broth (page 99).

If you cannot yet tolerate sour cream, substitute 1 large egg and 3 tbsp (45 mL) water, or 1 egg yolk and 6 tbsp (90 mL) Bone Broth.

Lamb Liver Pâté

Unless you are a homestead farmer breeding your own lambs, you might find precious lamb liver difficult to source. Check with a halal or kosher butcher, if there's one in your neighborhood, or try ordering it in advance from your supermarket's butcher department.

Tips

This pâté goes well with Cucumber Mint Salad (page 136).

This pâté is well suited for freezing, so you can stockpile it for future use. Wrap cooled pâtés well and freeze for up to 3 months. Let thaw in the refrigerator overnight.

You might choose to bake one pâté at a time and freeze the remaining pâtés unbaked. That way, you can quickly prepare a freshly baked pâté whenever you like. Don't forget to thaw it overnight in the refrigerator before baking!

Variation

If you cannot tolerate egg whites, replace the whole egg with 1 egg yolk and 3 tbsp (45 mL) Bone Broth (page 99).

- *Preheat oven to 340°F (170°C), with rack set in second-lowest position*
- *Meat grinder (see tip, page 126)*
- *Nut grinder (see box, page 75)*
- *3 small (1½- to 2-cup/375 to 500 mL) ovenproof pâté molds*

2 tbsp	cooking fat	30 mL
8 oz	mushrooms, chopped	250 g
1 lb	lamb liver	500 g
8 oz	lard from lamb, pork or veal	250 g
1	small onion, quartered	1
2½ oz	dried soaked hazelnuts (see page 74)	75 g
2	cloves garlic, minced (approx.)	2
1 tsp	dried thyme (approx.)	5 mL
1 tsp	crushed green peppercorns	5 mL
1 tsp	salt	5 mL
1	large egg, beaten	1
1 tbsp	Sour Cream (page 92)	15 mL
	Juice of ½ lemon (approx.)	

1. In a large skillet, melt cooking fat over medium-high heat. Add mushrooms and cook, stirring, for about 8 minutes or until lightly browned. Let cool.

2. Run liver and lard alternately with onion through meat grinder into a large bowl.

3. Grind hazelnuts to medium-fine flour.

4. Add nut flour, garlic, thyme, peppercorns, salt, egg, sour cream and lemon juice to liver mixture and stir well. Stir in mushrooms, including any liquid.

5. Form a small amount of the liver mixture into a ball. In skillet, fry meatball over medium heat until no longer pink inside. Taste meatball and adjust seasoning of remaining liver mixture with garlic, thyme, salt, pepper and/or lemon juice as desired.

6. Pack liver mixture into pâté molds, dividing equally.

7. Bake in preheated oven for 75 minutes or until a meat thermometer inserted in the center of a mold registers at least 160°F (71°C). Let pâtés cool in molds until lukewarm, or let cool completely and chill to serve cold.

Campfire Koftas

Makes 8 koftas
(1 per serving as a
snack; 2 per serving
as a meal)

When everyone else is
toasting hot dogs and
marshmallows, you can
grill some delicious koftas
instead. Prepare them in
your kitchen and bring
your kofta kit along to
the campfire.

Tips

Good choices for the herbs
and/or spices include thyme,
oregano, paprika and/or
curry powder.

Only embers are good for
this, not flames! Burnt food
is no good, especially for a
Gapster.

Keep an eye on the spit and
rotate the kofta often so it
turns out golden and crisp.

If you don't have a campfire
event to attend, you can grill
the koftas on a barbecue
grill instead.

- *8 toothpicks*
- *Lunch box or cooler*
- *Ice pack*

14 oz	ground meat (your choice)	400 g
1	small onion, finely chopped	1
½ tsp	salt	2 mL
	Freshly ground black pepper	
	Dried herbs and/or spices (your choice; see tip)	
½ to 1	large egg, beaten	½ to 1
2 tbsp	cooking fat	30 mL

To Serve

Thin slices bacon
Large lettuce leaves

1. In a medium bowl, combine meat, onion, salt, pepper, herbs and/or spices and enough egg just to moisten. Divide mixture into 8 equal portions and shape into oblong koftas.

2. In a large skillet, heat cooking fat over medium heat. Fry koftas, turning often, for about 10 minutes or until browned all over and a meat thermometer inserted in the thickest part of a kofta registers at least 160°F (71°C). Transfer to plate and let cool. (At this point, koftas can be refrigerated in an airtight container for up to 5 days or wrapped in packages of 1 or 2 and frozen in airtight containers or freezer bags for up to 3 months.)

3. *To pack and serve:* Wrap each kofta in a slice of bacon and fasten it with a toothpick. Place in a lunch box or cooler equipped with an ice pack. Rinse 1 lettuce leaf per kofta, pat dry and pack them as well.

4. At the campfire, find a fork-shaped twig with the two "tines" close together, strip off the bark and sharpen the ends to make a spit. Spear a kofta on the tines and grill over embers (see tip) until bacon is crisp.

5. Carefully remove kofta from spit and wrap in a lettuce leaf. You are now ready to enjoy a kofta in double wrap.

Vitello Tornado

*This recipe is inspired by
Italy's* vitello tonnato, *made of mayonnaise mixed with tuna and capers. Since most tuna, unfortunately, has a heavy metal content that is too high for Gapsters, my riff on the theme makes an excellent replacement.*

Tip

This dish is great as an appetizer or as part of a buffet or an especially festive luncheon.

• *Blender*

8 oz	braised veal (such as boneless rump roast or top round steak) or roast beef	250 g
	Veal Stock (page 102)	
1	large carrot, cooked	1
1	chunk cauliflower floret (about 5 oz/150 g), cooked	1
3 to 5 tbsp	freshly grated horseradish	45 to 75 mL
2 tbsp	Yogurt (page 92)	30 mL
1½ tbsp	cold-pressed olive oil	22 mL
1 tsp	peanut butter	5 mL
	Salt	

1. Cut veal into ultra-thin slices and arrange them individually on a serving platter or divide them among four plates. Drizzle each slice with a little stock.

2. In blender, combine carrot, cauliflower, 3 tbsp (45 mL) horseradish, yogurt, oil, peanut butter and salt to taste; purée until smooth. Taste and adjust seasoning with salt and horseradish as desired.

3. Place a spoonful of purée on each slice of meat and sprinkle with additional horseradish.

Chicken Nuggets

Makes 2 servings

Eat these tasty tidbits hot, lukewarm or cold, as tapas or in a lunch bag. Peanut Butter Sauce (page 185) is a delicious accompaniment.

Tips

Save the skin that you peel off the chicken and, in a dry skillet, fry it over medium-high heat in its own fat for 6 to 8 minutes or until golden and crisp. Sprinkle with salt and enjoy!

You can also use raw chicken; fry the coated pieces for about 10 minutes or until no longer pink inside.

- *Nut grinder (see box, page 75)*

1⅔ oz	dried soaked hazelnuts (see page 74)	50 g
4 tsp	coconut flour	20 mL
1 tbsp	curry powder	15 mL
	Salt and freshly ground black pepper	
1	large egg	1
2	small cooked chicken breasts (about 8 oz/250 g total), skin and bones removed, cut into bite-size pieces	2
	Cold-pressed coconut oil	

1. Grind hazelnuts to medium-fine flour and transfer to a shallow dish.

2. Add coconut flour and curry powder to nut flour, stirring to combine. Season with salt and pepper.

3. In another shallow dish, whisk egg until blended.

4. Working with one piece at a time, dip chicken first in egg, then in nut flour mixture, turning to coat. Discard any excess egg and nut flour mixture.

5. In a large skillet, heat a thick layer of coconut oil (4 to 6 tbsp/60 to 90 mL) over medium heat. Working in batches, fry chicken pieces for 2 to 3 minutes per side or until golden brown on all sides and chicken is heated through. Repeat with the remaining chicken pieces, adding coconut oil and adjusting heat as necessary between batches.

Variation

Raw cod may be substituted for the chicken; in step 5, fry until fish flakes easily when tested with a fork.

Club Salad

Makes 4 servings

*This luncheon treat is
so easy to prepare. Just
add the classic club
sandwich ingredients —
chicken, bacon and curry
mayonnaise — to crisp
salad greens, and voila!*

Tip

Tomato vinegar can be
purchased online. It adds
a wonderful umami flavor,
but if you don't have it on
hand, you can substitute a
good-quality no-sugar-added
balsamic vinegar.

8	slices bacon	8
2	cooked skin-on chicken breasts, bones removed	2
2/3 cup	Mayonnaise (page 187)	150 mL
1	clove garlic, minced	1
3 tbsp	chopped fresh parsley	45 mL
3 tbsp	chopped arugula	45 mL
1 tbsp	minced drained capers	15 mL
1 tsp	curry powder	5 mL
1/2 to 1 tsp	tomato vinegar	2 to 5 mL
	Salt and freshly ground black pepper	
4	handfuls green lettuce	4
8	cherry tomatoes, quartered	8

1. In a large skillet, in batches as necessary, fry bacon over medium-high heat until crisp. Using tongs, transfer bacon to a plate, reserving fat in skillet.

2. Peel skin off chicken breasts and set chicken aside. Add skin to bacon fat in skillet and fry over medium heat until browned and crisp. Let cool and break into small pieces as needed.

3. In a small bowl, combine mayonnaise, garlic, parsley, arugula, capers, curry powder and tomato vinegar to taste. Season to taste with salt and pepper.

4. Divide lettuce among 4 plates. Cut chicken into smaller pieces and arrange on top of lettuce. Spoon curry mayonnaise over chicken. Garnish with bacon, crisp chicken skin and cherry tomatoes.

Italian Salad

Makes 4 servings

This classic salad makes a wonderful accompaniment for fish cakes, chicken, cold tongue or ham.

Tip

If you use white asparagus in place of green, peel the stalks first and, in step 1, boil them for 6 to 7 minutes, depending on their thickness.

8 oz	asparagus, trimmed	250 g
3 to 5	carrots (about 8 oz/250 g total), finely diced	3 to 5
1 cup	frozen green peas	250 mL
1/2 cup	Mayonnaise (page 187)	125 mL
1 tbsp	Sour Cream (page 92)	15 mL
	Chopped fresh dill	
	Salt and freshly ground black pepper	

1. In a large pot of boiling salted water, boil asparagus for 5 minutes. Using tongs, transfer asparagus to a plate and let cool.

2. Add carrots to boiling water and boil for about 4 minutes or until slightly softened. Add green peas and boil for 2 minutes. Drain vegetables and let cool.

3. Cut asparagus into 3/4- to 1 1/2-inch (2 to 4 cm) pieces. Reserve some of the asparagus tips for garnish.

4. In a large bowl, combine mayonnaise, sour cream and dill to taste. Add carrots and green peas, stirring to coat, then stir in asparagus. Season to taste with salt and pepper. Serve garnished with reserved asparagus tips and more dill.

Beet Salad

Beets, especially raw beets, can be pretty tough for a Gapster to handle at first, but once your gut has healed a bit, you may enjoy this filling sweet-and-sour salad for lunch or as a side dish.

Tips

Use between 3 and 6 tbsp (45 and 90 mL) butter in step 1, depending on your preference and how much fat you need in your diet.

If you add a little Sour Cream (page 92) to the salad with the olive oil, it will taste even better.

	Butter, Clarified Butter (page 68) or coconut oil	
3	beets (about 14 oz/400 g total), peeled and coarsely grated	3
¼ cup	balsamic vinegar	60 mL
Pinch	salt	Pinch
1½ tbsp	dried soaked pine nuts (see page 74)	22 mL
2 tbsp	chopped fresh parsley	30 mL
1 to 2 tbsp	cold-pressed olive oil	15 to 30 mL

1. In a large skillet, melt desired amount of butter (see tip) over medium heat. Add beets and cook, stirring, for 3 minutes. Stir in vinegar and salt. Reduce heat to low, cover and simmer, stirring occasionally, for 30 minutes or until beets are very soft. Transfer to a bowl and let cool.

2. In a small dry skillet, toast pine nuts, stirring constantly, for about 3 minutes or until golden. Immediately transfer to a bowl and let cool.

3. Reserve some of the pine nuts and parsley for garnish. Add olive oil and remaining pine nuts and parsley to beets and let marinate at room temperature for 10 to 30 minutes.

4. Transfer beet mixture to a serving bowl and garnish with reserved pine nuts and parsley.

Brussels Sprout and Apple Salad

Makes 4 servings

According to the recommendations for the GAPS diet, fruit should mainly be enjoyed between meals because of how it interferes with the digestion of "real food." There are, however, two exceptions to this guideline: lemons and apples go well with meals.

Tip

If you are far enough along in the diet that you can tolerate semicooked Brussels sprouts, skip step 2 and, instead, slice them and blanch them quickly in lightly salted water before patting them dry and mixing them into the salad.

¼ cup	cold-pressed olive oil	60 mL
1 tbsp	apple cider vinegar	15 mL
1 tsp	liquid honey	5 mL
20	Brussels sprouts, outer leaves removed	20
½ oz	dried soaked almonds (see page 74), coarsely chopped	15 g
1	large apple	1

1. In a small bowl, whisk together oil, vinegar and honey.

2. In a saucepan of boiling lightly salted water, boil Brussels sprouts for about 8 minutes or until tender. Drain and let cool.

3. In a small dry skillet, toast almonds, stirring constantly, for about 5 minutes or until lightly browned. Immediately transfer to a bowl and let cool.

4. Thinly slice Brussels sprouts and dice apple, placing them in a large bowl as you go. Add dressing and toss to coat.

5. Transfer salad to a serving bowl and sprinkle with toasted almonds.

Cucumber Mint Salad

Makes 4 servings

This refreshing salad is exceptionally good when paired with lamb.

Tips

Tomato vinegar can be purchased online. It adds a wonderful umami flavor, but if you don't have it on hand, you can substitute a good-quality no-sugar-added balsamic vinegar.

Omit the raw onion if you cannot yet tolerate it.

Marinade

1	small clove garlic, minced	1
2 tbsp	cold-pressed olive oil	30 mL
1 tsp	raw honey	5 mL
1/2 tsp	Dijon mustard	2 mL
1/2 tsp	tomato vinegar	2 mL
Pinch	salt	Pinch

Salad

1	cucumber (about 6 inches/15 cm long), finely diced	1
2	slices onion, chopped	2
30	fresh mint leaves, chopped	30

1. *Marinade:* In a large bowl, whisk together garlic, oil, honey, mustard, vinegar and salt.

2. *Salad:* Add cucumber, onion and mint to marinade and toss to coat. Let stand for 15 minutes before serving.

Root Vegetable Patties

Makes 8 patties

These veggie patties are great as a quick snack, on their own in a lunch bag or with hummus or guacamole (page 139).

Tips

Sesame flour is available online and at some well-stocked health food stores.

You may, of course, add any spices and herbs you tolerate to the root vegetable mixture.

7 oz	Mashed Root Vegetables (page 181)	200 g
1	large egg	1
1	clove garlic, minced	1
1 tbsp	sesame flour	15 mL
	Salt and freshly ground black pepper	
1/4 cup	cooking fat	60 mL

1. In a bowl, whisk mashed root vegetables with egg and garlic. Stir in sesame flour and salt and pepper to taste.

2. In a large skillet, melt cooking fat over medium heat. Working in batches, drop dollops of mashed vegetables the size of small pancakes into hot skillet, spacing them apart. Fry for about 10 minutes, turning once, until golden brown on both sides, adjusting heat as necessary to prevent patties from burning or falling apart. Using a slotted spatula, transfer patties to a plate. Repeat with the remaining mashed vegetables, adding fat and adjusting heat as necessary between batches.

Potato Salad for the Transition Diet

Makes 4 servings

This is a meal in its own right, but it's also very nice with Meatballs (page 157).

Tips

The eggs may be omitted if you are serving the salad as an accompaniment to a heavier and more nourishing dish.

Freshly made sour cream tends to be runnier, so in step 5, just add the minimum amount to avoid a wet salad; if your sour cream has had time to thicken, add more for better flavor and texture and more probiotics.

Be sure to wait to try this recipe until you have followed the GAPS nutritional protocol long enough to recover fully and have had at least 6 months of good health. Introduce it gradually and carefully, keeping in mind that, depending on the severity of your health problem, you may never be able to reintroduce potatoes into your diet.

1¼ lbs	new potatoes	625 g
8 oz	frozen green peas	250 g
⅔ oz	dried soaked pine nuts (see page 74)	20 g
4	large eggs	4
½ cup	Oil and Vinegar Dressing (page 192)	125 mL
¼ to ⅔ cup	Sour Cream (page 92)	60 to 150 mL
	Salt and freshly ground black pepper	
½	small onion, finely chopped	½
½	cucumber, diced	½
4	tomatoes, cut into quarters, divided	4

1. Place potatoes in a saucepan and add cold water to cover. Bring to a boil over high heat. Reduce heat and boil gently until potatoes are tender. Let cool, then peel and slice potatoes.

2. Place green peas in a small saucepan and add cold water to cover. Bring to a boil over high heat. Drain and let cool.

3. In a small dry skillet, toast pine nuts, stirring constantly, for about 3 minutes or until golden. Immediately transfer to a bowl and let cool.

4. Place eggs in a saucepan and add cold water to cover. Bring to a boil over high heat. Boil for 5 minutes or until the outer edges of the whites and yolks are hard and the center of the yolks are soft. Drain and chill in cold water, then peel eggs and cut in half.

5. In a large bowl, whisk together dressing and desired amount of sour cream (see tip). Season to taste with salt and pepper. Stir in green peas, onion and cucumber, then add potatoes and half the tomatoes, tossing gently to coat.

6. Transfer potato salad to a serving bowl and garnish with pine nuts, eggs and the remaining tomatoes.

Falafels

These fried bean balls go well with tomato soup or a salad, and they are great as part of a buffet or for packing in a lunch bag.

Tips

Make sure to prepare the beans properly, as described on page 72. Keep in mind that, even after this preparation, some people may find them difficult or impossible to digest.

Sesame flour is available online and at some well-stocked health food stores.

Choose a good-quality brand of unflavored gelatin powder made from grass-fed animals, such as Great Lakes or Vital Protein. For more information, see page 55.

Use between 4 and 6 tbsp (60 and 90 mL) cooking fat in step 4, depending on your preference and how much fat you need in your diet.

If you are using an electric stove, you may need to use medium-low or medium heat in step 4 to get enough heat to cook the falafels.

• *Blender*

2 tbsp	butter or other cooking fat	30 mL
1/3	small onion, coarsely chopped	1/3
1²/₃ cups	cooked white beans (page 72)	400 mL
1 or 2	cloves garlic	1 or 2
2 tbsp	sesame flour	30 mL
2 tbsp	chopped fresh cilantro	30 mL
1/2 to 1 tsp	ground cumin	2 to 5 mL
1/4 to 1/2 tsp	ground coriander	1 to 2 mL
1/2 tsp	salt	2 mL
Pinch	cayenne pepper	Pinch
1	large egg	1
1¹/₂ tsp	freshly squeezed lemon juice	7 mL
2 tsp	unflavored gelatin powder	10 mL
	Animal fat or Clarified Butter (page 68)	

1. In a small saucepan, melt 2 tbsp (30 mL) butter over medium heat. Add onion and cook, stirring, for 5 minutes or until softened. Let cool slightly.

2. In blender, combine beans, garlic to taste, sesame flour, cilantro, cumin and coriander to taste, salt, cayenne, egg and lemon juice; blend until smooth. Add onion and blend until consistency is smooth and creamy.

3. Transfer bean mixture to a bowl. Sprinkle with gelatin while stirring. Mix well and let stand for 5 minutes. Shape into 14 balls.

4. In a large skillet, melt desired amount of animal fat over low heat (see tips). Cook falafels for 15 minutes, turning occasionally, until golden brown on all sides, adjusting heat as necessary so they don't burn. Be careful to maintain their round shape.

Variation

If you have an ebelskiver pan, you can use it to cook the falafels. Omit the gelatin and cook the falafels in two batches, increasing the cooking time for each batch to about 18 minutes.

White Bean Hummus

Makes 4 servings

*Converting hummus into
a GAPS-friendly recipe
is quite easy: you simply
use well-prepared white
beans instead of chickpeas.
Hummus goes well with
olives, carrots, celery,
red pepper and cucumber.*

Tip

Wait until you are well into
the diet before eating beans,
and start with small amounts.
Make sure to prepare them
properly, as described on
page 72.

* **Blender**

1²⁄₃ cups	cooked white beans (see page 72)	400 mL
¼ cup	cold-pressed olive oil (approx.)	60 mL
1	clove garlic	1
2 tbsp	sesame seeds, toasted (page 74)	30 mL
½ tsp	ground cumin	2 mL
½ tsp	salt	2 mL
Pinch	cayenne pepper	Pinch
	Juice of ½ lemon	

1. In blender, process beans and oil until beans are finely
   chopped. Add garlic, sesame seeds, cumin, salt, cayenne
   and lemon juice; process until smooth, adding more oil
   as needed for a smooth consistency. Taste and adjust
   seasoning as desired with a little of this or that.

2. Transfer to an airtight container and store in the
   refrigerator for up to 3 days.

Guacamole

Makes 6 to 8 servings

*Serve guacamole as a side
dish for lunch or as a dip
with raw vegetables and
Sesame Crisps (page 199).*

Variation

If you omit the lemon
juice and cayenne
pepper, you can enjoy
this recipe from stage 4
of the intro diet.

4	ripe avocados	4
1	clove garlic, minced	1
2 tbsp	cold-pressed olive oil	30 mL
1 tbsp	Sour Cream (page 92)	15 mL
	Juice of ½ lemon	
2	large ripe tomatoes	2
Pinch	cayenne pepper (optional)	Pinch
	Salt and freshly ground black pepper	

1. In a bowl, mash avocados with garlic, olive oil, sour cream
   and lemon juice.

2. Cut tomatoes in half, remove seeds and finely dice firm
   tomato flesh.

3. Add tomatoes and cayenne (if using) to guacamole.
   Season to taste with salt and pepper, stirring gently.

Dinners

Hearty Chicken Stew

Makes 4 to 6 servings

Who would have thought that a fairly simple casserole like this one could be not only nourishing but also healing?

Variation

Hearty Fish Stew: Substitute Fish Stock (page 103) and fish for the chicken stock and chicken.

2 cups	Chicken Stock (page 102)	500 mL
	Salt	
6	carrots, sliced	6
1	large onion, sliced	1
2	zucchini or yellow summer squash, cubed	2
1	red bell pepper, sliced	1
2½ lbs	meat (with skin) from 1 cooked chicken, cut into bite-size pieces	1.25 kg
4	cloves garlic, finely minced	4
1 cup	frozen green peas, thawed	250 mL
1 tsp	butter, Clarified Butter (page 68) or coconut oil	5 mL
	Freshly ground black pepper	

1. In a medium pot, bring lightly salted stock to a boil over medium-high heat. Add carrots and onion; reduce heat and simmer for 15 minutes.

2. Add zucchini and red pepper; simmer for 10 minutes or until vegetables are very tender.

3. Stir in chicken, garlic, peas, butter, and salt and pepper to taste; simmer until chicken is heated through.

Creating Your Own Stews for the Intro Diet, Stage 2, and On

When you have reached stage 2 of the intro diet, you may eat stews or casseroles made with the meat or fish from which you made stock, along with your favorite stage-appropriate vegetables (see lists, pages 21–23). You can keep creating and enjoying dishes like these all the way through the diet!

Starting with stage 2, you should be adding cooking fat such as clarified butter, butter or coconut oil to your recipes, but do not use it for frying until stage 4.

Vegetables should be cooked until they are very tender, and you should stay away from vegetables with coarse fiber, such as rutabaga, cauliflower stems and broccoli stems. For flavor, add finely chopped fresh herbs, such as parsley, chives, dill, basil, cilantro, watercress and chervil.

Turkey, Mushroom and Spinach Stew

Makes 5 to 6 servings

If you can get hold of a whole turkey, you can divide it into quite a few parts and save them in the freezer for future meals. The easiest part of the turkey to use for this stew is the breast, but really, you can use any turkey meat you like.

Tip

Choose organic frozen spinach with no additives. You don't need to chop the spinach, but you can if you like.

1¾ lbs	skin-on boneless turkey breast, cut into 1-inch (2.5 cm) cubes	875 g
5	cloves garlic, sliced	5
1	large onion, coarsely chopped	1
1 tsp	salt	5 mL
1 tsp	freshly ground black pepper	5 mL
2 cups	Chicken Stock (page 102)	500 mL
1 tbsp	apple cider vinegar	15 mL
1 lb	mushrooms, sliced	500 g
8 oz	frozen whole spinach, thawed and patted dry	250 g
	Chopped fresh parsley	

1. In a large pot, combine turkey, garlic, onion, salt, pepper, stock and vinegar; bring to a simmer over medium heat. Simmer for 15 minutes.

2. Add mushrooms and simmer for 10 minutes or until vegetables are very tender and turkey is no longer pink inside.

3. Stir in spinach and simmer for 5 minutes or until spinach is heated through. Serve sprinkled with parsley.

Veal Stew

This stew is similar to a fricassee but without the sautéing step. Because the meat isn't browned and egg yolk is a key component of the white sauce, it fits nicely into stage 2 of the intro diet.

Tips

You might want to let your butcher do the work of cutting the veal into cubes for you.

Save the egg whites for baking recipes. Store them in an airtight container in the refrigerator for up to 3 days or in the freezer for up to 6 months.

Publisher's note: This recipe contains egg yolks that are not fully cooked. Although raw eggs are considered nourishing in the GAPS diet, they may contain salmonella (see sidebar, page 22). If you prefer to err on the side of caution, use the yolks from pasteurized in-shell eggs, if they are available in your area. Otherwise, you may want to omit the egg yolks and skip steps 4 and 6, serving the stew as is after step 5. Note that, while pasteurized eggs are not part of the GAPS nutritional protocol, food safety must be your first priority.

2½ lbs	boneless veal stewing meat (such as arm or blade roast), cut into 1½- by 1-inch (4 by 2.5 cm) cubes	1.25 kg
5 cups	water	1.25 L
2 tsp	salt	10 mL
4	bay leaves	4
1 tsp	black peppercorns	5 mL
4 cups	chopped celery root (1½- by 1-inch/ 4 by 2.5 cm chunks)	1 L
3½ cups	sliced onions	875 mL
3 cups	chopped carrots (1½- by 1-inch/ 4 by 2.5 cm chunks)	750 mL
2 cups	frozen green peas, thawed	500 mL
½ to 1 cup	fresh dill, finely chopped	125 to 250 mL
	Salt and freshly ground black pepper	
4	large egg yolks (see tip)	4

1. In a large pot, combine veal, water and salt; bring to a boil over medium heat. Skim off and discard any foam.

2. Add bay leaves and peppercorns. Reduce heat to low, cover and simmer for about 1 hour or until meat is almost tender.

3. Stir in celery root, onions and carrots; cover and simmer for 20 minutes or until vegetables are tender. Stir in peas, cover and simmer for 5 minutes. Discard bay leaves.

4. Using a ladle, scoop about 1 cup (250 mL) stock from the pot and transfer to a small bowl; let cool slightly.

5. Stir chopped dill to taste into the pot and season to taste with salt and pepper; simmer, stirring, for 1 minute. Remove from heat.

6. Whisk egg yolks into the bowl of lukewarm stock. Spoon stew into serving bowls and pour yolky sauce over top.

Lamb and Cabbage Stew

Makes 4 to 6 servings

This recipe is a real treat: easy to prepare, filling and satisfying!

Tips

Ask your butcher to coarsely chop the shoulder meat and bone, as for goulash.

You may also cook this dish in a large pot on the stovetop. Let it simmer over low heat for a couple of hours, stirring occasionally.

Reserve the lamb bones after cooking to make Bone Broth (page 99).

- **Preheat oven to 340°F (170°C)**
- **Roasting pan or large ovenproof pot**

5	carrots, chopped	5
2	leeks (white and light green parts only), sliced	2
2	slices celery root, chopped	2
1	cabbage (about 2 lbs/1 kg), shredded	1
8 to 10	cloves garlic, cut in half	8 to 10
4 lbs	chopped bone-in lamb shoulder (see tip)	2 kg
	Salt and freshly ground black pepper	
4 cups	Chicken or Veal Stock (page 102)	1 L
	Chopped fresh parsley	

1. In roasting pan, combine carrots, leeks, celery root and cabbage. Arrange garlic to taste on top. Place lamb on top of vegetables and season with salt and pepper. Pour stock over top. Cover with lid or foil.

2. Roast in preheated oven for about 2 hours or until lamb and vegetables are very tender. Serve with a bowl of parsley to sprinkle over top.

Meatball Stew with Spinach and Celery Root

Makes 4 to 6 servings		

This stew is really nice at any time of year, and you can use any type of ground meat you prefer.

Tips

Choose organic frozen spinach with no additives.

Using frozen spinach saves you a lot of prep time, but of course you can use fresh spinach instead! For this recipe, you'll need a large handful. Rinse it, remove any tough stalks and coarsely chop it before adding it to the stew.

Use between 1 tsp (5 mL) and 2 tbsp (30 mL) cooking fat in step 6, depending on your preference and how much fat you need in your diet.

$2\frac{1}{2}$ to $3\frac{1}{4}$ cups	Chicken or Veal Stock (page 102)	625 to 800 mL
1	large carrot, grated	1
$\frac{1}{2}$	onion, finely chopped	$\frac{1}{2}$
$\frac{1}{2}$ to 1	celery root, diced	$\frac{1}{2}$ to 1
1 lb	full-fat ground meat	500 g
3	cloves garlic, minced	3
	Salt and freshly ground black pepper	
14 oz	frozen spinach, thawed, squeezed dry and coarsely chopped	400 g
	Cooking fat	

1. In a large saucepan, bring $2\frac{1}{2}$ cups (625 mL) stock to a boil over medium-high heat. Add carrot and onion, reduce heat and simmer for about 5 minutes or until vegetables are softened.

2. Using a sieve, remove vegetables from stock, transfer to a large bowl and let cool.

3. To the stock, add celery root to taste and simmer for 15 minutes or until almost tender.

4. Meanwhile, add ground meat and garlic to carrot and onion, season with salt and pepper, and mix to combine. Form into small meatballs, about 2 inches (5 cm) in diameter, squeezing them well.

5. Add meatballs to the stock, add more stock if needed to cover meatballs and simmer for 15 minutes or until meatballs are no longer pink inside and celery root is very tender.

6. Stir in spinach and cooking fat (see tip); simmer for 5 minutes.

Oven-Baked Mackerel with Apple Compote

Makes 4 servings

Fatty fish like mackerel taste great with something sour and sharp to accompany it. A not-too-sweet apple compote made with fiery chiles fits the bill nicely.

Tip

You can add more fish fillets if you need more than 4 servings. Bake for an additional 8 to 10 minutes.

- **Preheat oven to 340°F (170°C), with rack set in middle position**
- **Ovenproof dish**

| 4 | skin-on mackerel fillets (or 8 herring fillets), thawed if frozen | 4 |
| 3 cups | Spicy Apple Compote (page 170) Salt and freshly ground black pepper | 750 mL |

1. Rinse fish under cold running water, cut off fins if necessary and pat dry.

2. Pour compote into ovenproof dish and place mackerel on top, skin side up, overlapping if necessary. Season with salt and pepper.

3. Bake in preheated oven for 15 minutes or until fish flakes easily when tested with a fork.

Fried Herring

8	herring fillets, thawed if frozen	8
1 or 2	large eggs	1 or 2
1 cup	sesame flour	250 mL
	Salt and freshly ground black pepper	
	Clarified Butter (page 68)	

Makes 3 to 4 servings

The small Scandinavian country of Denmark has survived thanks to this recipe! Because herring was the most plentiful fatty fish from the sea, Danes traditionally ate it for breakfast, lunch and dinner. Other small fatty fish can be used in place of herring.

Tips

Keep the fried herring fillets warm by placing them in a small dish on top of a pot of simmering vegetables.

You don't need eggs and sesame flour, but the fish is even more delicious with the coating.

Sesame flour is available online and at some well-stocked health food stores.

1. Rinse fish under cold running water, cut off fins if necessary and pat dry.

2. In a shallow dish, whisk 1 egg until blended. In another shallow dish, combine sesame flour, salt and pepper. One at a time, dip fish fillets in egg mixture, then dredge in flour mixture. Place on a plate. Whisk another egg if needed to coat fillets. Discard any excess egg and flour mixture.

3. In a skillet, heat a thick layer of clarified butter over medium heat. Working in batches, fry fish fillets for 2 to 3 minutes per side or until golden brown on both sides and fish flakes easily when tested with a fork.

Baked Salmon

Makes 3 to 4 servings

Baked salmon is easy to prepare and is great for lunch or supper or on a party buffet table.

Tips

The number of servings depends on the size of the salmon.

Mushroom Fish Sauce (page 183) or Pesto (page 191) goes well with this dish.

- *Preheat oven to 350°F (180°C), with rack set in second-lowest position*
- *Large baking dish, greased*

1	wild salmon fillet (about 1½ lbs/750 g)	1
1 to 2	cloves garlic, finely chopped	1 to 2
	Grated zest of ½ lemon	
	Salt and freshly ground black pepper	
	Butter, cut into small pieces	

1. Place salmon, skin side down, in prepared dish. Scatter garlic and lemon zest over top. Season with salt and pepper and top with pats of butter.

2. Bake in preheated oven for about 20 minutes or until fish is opaque and flakes easily when tested with a fork.

Variation

If you omit the lemon zest, the recipe can be enjoyed from stage 4 of the intro diet.

Fish Fillets with Spinach

Makes 4 servings

If you or your kids don't like fish because of the bones, this is the recipe for you! It's just nice white fish, spicy spinach and no bones.

Tip

You may, of course, omit the spinach and spices and just make steamed fish with butter.

	Butter or Clarified Butter (page 68)	
1	onion, chopped	1
1 tsp	ground turmeric	5 mL
1/2 tsp	ground coriander	2 mL
Pinch	cayenne pepper	Pinch
8 oz	frozen whole spinach, thawed, squeezed dry and coarsely chopped	250 g
8 to 12	thin skinless white fish fillets, such as sole, cod or tilapia (about 1 1/2 lbs/ 750 kg total)	8 to 12
	Salt and freshly ground black pepper	

1. In a large skillet, melt a thick layer of butter over medium-low heat. Add onion, turmeric, coriander and cayenne, stirring well. Cover and simmer for 10 minutes.

2. Stir in spinach. Arrange fish fillets on top, overlapping as necessary, seasoning each fillet with salt and pepper as you layer. Cover and steam for 5 minutes or until fish is opaque and flakes easily when tested with a fork.

Fish Cakes

Makes 4 servings
(about 16 cakes)

Serve these fish cakes with any type of vegetable or green lettuce. They pair well with many different cold sauces, such as Ravigote Sauce (page 189), Rémoulade (page 189) or Green Sauce (page 188).

Tips

Use between 2 and 4 tbsp (30 and 60 mL) cooking fat in step 1, depending on your preference and how much fat you need in your diet.

Make sure to prepare the beans properly, as described on page 72. Keep in mind that, even after this preparation, some people may find them difficult or impossible to digest.

These cakes are more fragile and burn more easily than fish cakes that contain flour, so don't use a higher heat than medium-low.

Make more fish cakes than you need for dinner and freeze some for future lunches.

- *Blender*
- *Electric mixer*

	Cooking fat	
1	small onion, chopped	1
1¼ lbs	skinless pollock or cod fillets, cut into small pieces	625 g
⅔ cup	cooked white beans (page 72)	150 mL
½ to 1 tsp	salt	2 to 5 mL
2	large eggs, separated	2

1. In a skillet, melt desired amount of cooking fat (see tip) over low heat. Add onion and cook, stirring often, for about 10 minutes or until very soft.

2. Transfer onion to blender and purée until smooth. Add fish, beans, salt and egg yolks; process until fish and beans are finely chopped and mixture is paste-like. Transfer to a bowl.

3. In a small bowl, using electric mixer, beat egg whites until stiff.

4. Using a spatula, gently fold one-quarter of the egg whites into fish mixture to make it light. Fold in another quarter until blended, then fold in the remaining whites.

5. In the same skillet, melt ¼ cup (60 mL) cooking fat over medium-low heat. In batches as necessary, spoon fish mixture into skillet, using the desired amount of batter per cake and spacing cakes apart. Fry for about 8 minutes per side or until cakes are golden brown and hot in the center, adjusting heat as necessary between batches to prevent burning.

Variation

If you substitute 3 tbsp (45 mL) nut or seed flour for the white beans, this recipe can be enjoyed from stage 4 of the intro diet.

Fish Lasagna

Makes 4 servings

This wonderful dish may take some time to prepare, but I promise you will enjoy it!

Tip

Serve the lasagna with a salad or baked root vegetables.

- *Preheat oven to 350°F (180°C), with rack set in second-lowest position*
- *13- by 9-inch (33 by 23 cm) glass baking dish*

	Cooking fat	
4	large eggs	4
3/4 cup	Sour Cream (page 92)	175 mL
1/4 tsp	grated lemon zest	1 mL
	Freshly ground black pepper	
4	zucchini or yellow summer squash, cut lengthwise into very thin slices	4
1 lb	skinless white fish fillets, cut into bite-size pieces	500 g
2 1/2 tbsp	Pesto (page 191)	37 mL
10	Marinated Sun-Dried Tomatoes (page 197), thinly shredded	10
1/2 cup	shredded Swiss cheese	60 g

1. Place a large pat of cooking fat in baking dish. Place in preheated oven for about 3 minutes to melt fat.

2. In a bowl, whisk eggs until blended; whisk in sour cream, lemon zest and pepper (this is the white sauce).

3. Brush melted fat in dish to evenly coat bottom and sides. Arrange ingredients in layers in the following order: zucchini, white sauce, fish, small dots of pesto and shredded tomatoes. End with a layer of sauce garnished with pesto and shredded tomatoes. Sprinkle cheese on top.

4. Bake lasagna for 50 minutes or until bubbling hot, zucchini is tender and fish is opaque and flakes easily when tested with a fork.

Variation

For a luxury version, use deveined peeled shrimp along with the fish.

Thai-Style Chicken Legs

Who would have thought you could eat such a delicious, satisfying dish as part of a diet? It pairs especially well with Mushrooms with Spinach (page 177). Enjoy!

Tip

You can get coconut water either directly from a juicy coconut or by soaking 3 tbsp (45 mL) coconut flour overnight in ¾ cup (175 mL) water.

4	chicken leg quarters	4
	Salt and freshly ground black pepper	
2 to 3 tsp	curry powder	10 to 15 mL
	Coconut oil	
4	carrots, diced	4
1	onion, finely chopped	1
1	1¼-inch (3 cm) piece gingerroot, grated	1
2	cloves garlic, chopped	2
¾ cup	coconut water or coconut milk	175 mL
½ cup	Bone Broth (page 99)	125 mL
	Juice of 1 lime	
	Chopped fresh cilantro	

1. Rub chicken legs with salt, pepper and curry powder.

2. In a large skillet, heat a thin layer of coconut oil over medium-high heat. In batches as necessary, add chicken legs, skin side down, and cook, turning once, until browned on both sides. Transfer to a plate.

3. Reduce heat to medium and add carrots, onion and ginger to skillet, along with more coconut oil, if needed; cook, stirring, for about 10 minutes or until softened.

4. Stir in garlic, coconut water, broth and lime juice. Place chicken on top. Reduce heat to low, cover and simmer for about 30 minutes or until juices run clear when chicken is pierced.

5. Serve with a bowl of cilantro to sprinkle on top.

Apple Pork

Makes 4 servings

Organic pork fat provides equal amounts of monounsaturated and saturated fatty acids, but even more importantly, it delivers taste, juiciness and crispness! Serve this dish with well-cooked vegetables such as cauliflower, pointed cabbage, Brussels sprouts, carrots or green peas, or with fermented vegetables such as sauerkraut.

Tip

Store any cut-off non-bruised apple parts for your next batch of juice.

- *Preheat oven to 200°F (100°C)*
- *Ovenproof platter*

12 to 16	thick slices side pork	12 to 16
	Salt	
1	onion, sliced	1
3	large cooking apples, quartered	3

1. In a large skillet over medium-high heat, fry pork slices in batches, sprinkling with salt and turning once, for about 20 minutes or until crisp. Transfer fried pork to the ovenproof platter and keep warm in preheated oven. Pour excess fat from the pan into a bowl between batches and reserve this gold for future frying and baking. Leave the fat from the last batch in the pan.

2. Add onion to skillet, reduce heat to medium-low and cook, stirring, for about 5 minutes or until almost soft. Add apples, cover and cook for about 10 minutes or until tender. Pour onion and apples over pork slices.

Sweet-and-Sour Pork

Makes 6 servings

This is really just a GAPS-friendly version of spareribs. Bake or grill them in the oven, or bring marinated ready-to-grill pork along on your next picnic.

Tips

Plan ahead and start marinating the pork the night before.

Sauerkraut (page 84 or 86) is a great accompaniment to any kind of pork dish.

6 tbsp	tomato purée	90 mL
3 tbsp	liquid honey	45 mL
	Juice of ½ lemon	
1 tsp	salt	5 mL
	Freshly ground black pepper	
24	thick slices side pork	24

1. In a bowl, combine tomato purée, honey, lemon juice, salt and pepper to taste. Add pork and stir to coat. Cover and refrigerate for at least 1 hour or up to 1 day.

2. Preheat oven to 350°F (180°C), with rack set in second-lowest position.

3. Transfer pork to a roasting pan, arranging it in layers as necessary, and cover with marinade.

4. Bake for 1 hour, turning once, until pork is very tender.

Variation

In place of the sliced side pork, use 2 slabs of pork side ribs or spareribs.

Slow-Braised Pork Hocks

Makes 3 servings

If you need a satisfyingly fatty meal, this is it! When you have the time, make pork the South German way — you won't be disappointed.

Tip

Sauerkraut (page 84 or 86) is made to accompany pork hocks, as is unsweetened apple cider.

- *Preheat oven to 325°F (160°C)*
- *Baking dish*
- *Kitchen string (optional)*

2	pork hocks (each about 2 lbs/1 kg)	2
	Salt	
1	onion, cut into quarters	1
1	carrot, cut in half	1

1. Using a sharp knife, score pork hocks in a diamond pattern. Rub plenty of salt all over the hocks.

2. Place onion and carrot in baking dish. Place hocks on top. (You may tie them together with string to make them stand upright.) Pour a little water into bottom of dish.

3. Bake in preheated oven for 4 to 6 hours, adding more water if necessary during baking to keep hocks moist and basting hocks occasionally, until meat is very tender and falling off the bones.

Meatballs

Makes 4 to 5 servings		

Once you are familiar with this basic recipe, you can start to improvise: add your favorite spices or herbs, and use any type of ground meat, so long as it is not lean. Serve the meatballs with well-cooked leeks, cabbage, winter or summer squash, carrots or peas, with Cauliflower Couscous (page 174), Beet Salad (page 134) or a green salad, or, when you're transitioning out of the GAPS diet, with Potato Salad for the Transition Diet (page 137). Try them with Soft-Curd Cheese with Herbs (page 196) or even homemade Ketchup (page 190). They're also nice cold.

Tips

Use between 2 and 4 tbsp (30 and 60 mL) cooking fat in step 1 and in step 3, depending on your preference and how much fat you need in your diet.

Cook plenty so you have enough left over for lunch the next day. Let meatballs cool and store in an airtight container in the refrigerator for up to 3 days.

	Cooking fat	
1	onion, chopped	1
½	zucchini or yellow summer squash (about 4 oz/125 g), coarsely grated	½
1 lb	ground pork, veal, lamb or beef (not lean)	500 g
1	large clove garlic, minced	1
½ tsp	dried thyme	2 mL
1	large egg	1
½ tsp	salt	2 mL
	Freshly ground black pepper	

1. In a skillet, melt desired amount of cooking fat (see tip) over low heat. Add onion and zucchini; cook, stirring, for 5 minutes or until almost tender. Let cool.

2. In a bowl, combine ground meat, garlic, thyme, egg, salt and pepper. Add onion mixture and stir to combine. Scoop up 1-tbsp (15 mL) portions of meat mixture and form into balls.

3. In the same skillet, heat desired amount of cooking fat over medium heat. Add meatballs and fry for about 5 minutes per side or until no longer pink inside.

Variation

Replace the zucchini with a couple of spoonfuls of Baked Pumpkin or Squash (page 77) or, if you can tolerate them, mashed cooked beans or lentils (page 72 or 73).

Bolognese Sauce

Makes 8 servings			

This meat sauce is wonderful served over Carrot and Zucchini Spaghetti (page 182), with freshly grated Parmesan cheese sprinkled over top.

Tips

You may substitute 4 large stalks celery for celery root.

Tomato vinegar can be purchased online. It adds a wonderful umami flavor, but if you don't have it on hand, you can substitute a good-quality no-sugar-added balsamic vinegar.

If you prefer a thicker sauce, use less broth in step 3; if you prefer a thinner sauce, use more.

	Cooking fat	
2 lbs	ground veal or beef	1 kg
1	large onion, finely chopped	1
4	carrots, finely diced	4
1/4	celery root (about 10 oz/300 g), finely diced	1/4
4	cloves garlic, minced	4
2 tbsp	tomato purée	30 mL
1/2 tsp	dried thyme	2 mL
1 tsp	salt	5 mL
	Freshly ground black pepper	
2 cups	crushed tomatoes (from a jar)	500 mL
1 2/3 to 2 cups	Bone Broth (page 99)	400 to 500 mL
1 1/2 tsp	tomato vinegar (optional)	7 mL

1. In a large pot, melt a thin layer of cooking fat over medium-high heat. Add one-third of the ground meat and cook, stirring and breaking it up, until no longer pink. Using a slotted spoon, transfer browned meat to a bowl. Brown the remaining meat in two more batches, adding more cooking fat and adjusting the heat as needed between batches.

2. Reduce heat to medium-low, add onion and cook, stirring, for about 5 minutes or until translucent. Add carrots and celery root; cook, stirring, for about 4 minutes or until softened. Add garlic, tomato purée, thyme, salt, and pepper to taste.

3. Stir in crushed tomatoes and desired amount of broth (see tip). Return meat and any accumulated juices to pot and bring to a simmer. Reduce heat to low, cover and simmer, stirring occasionally, for 50 to 55 minutes or until sauce is thickened and flavors are blended. Stir in tomato vinegar (if using).

Fried Liver with Onions and Mushrooms

Makes 4 servings

This is an old-fashioned recipe that deserves a revival. Serve it with well-cooked cauliflower, pointed cabbage or broccoli, Mashed Root Vegetables (page 181) or Oven-Baked Vegetables (page 180).

Tips

Use between 2 and 4 tbsp (30 and 60 mL) cooking fat in step 2 and in step 5, depending on your preference and how much fat you need in your diet.

Try sprinkling fried bacon cubes over the liver when serving.

1¼ lbs	veal, beef or lamb liver	625 g
	Salt and freshly ground black pepper	
1 tbsp	cold-pressed olive oil	15 mL
	Juice of ½ lemon	
	Clarified Butter (page 68) or animal fat	
2	onions, sliced	2
½ tsp	dried thyme	2 mL
1 tbsp	no-sugar-added balsamic vinegar	15 mL
8 oz	mushrooms, halved	250 g
2	cloves garlic, minced	2
2 tbsp	Sour Cream (page 92)	30 mL

1. Remove membrane from liver and cut meat into ½-inch (1 cm) thick slices. Transfer to a plate in a single layer and sprinkle with salt, pepper, olive oil and lemon juice. Set aside to marinate at room temperature.

2. In a medium skillet, melt desired amount of cooking fat (see tip) over medium heat. Add onions, thyme and vinegar; cook, stirring often, for 10 to 15 minutes or until golden and soft.

3. Meanwhile, in a large skillet, melt 2 tbsp (30 mL) cooking fat over medium heat. Add mushrooms and cook, stirring, for about 10 minutes or until tender.

4. Add mushrooms to onions (reserve large skillet). Add garlic and cook, stirring, for 2 minutes. Stir in sour cream. Reduce heat to low, cover and simmer for 5 minutes.

5. Return large skillet to high heat and melt desired amount of cooking fat. Working in batches, fry liver slices over medium-high heat, turning often, for about 4 minutes or to desired doneness.

6. Spoon onion mixture onto plates and top with liver slices.

GAPS-Friendly Pizza with a Crispy Crust

Makes 4 servings

This easy technique produces a crispy pizza crust! Plus, it incorporates gelatin, a medicinal food. You can, of course, use many different toppings, as long as they are GAPS-friendly. Try it with air-dried ham, lightly fried eggplant slices, shellfish, anchovies, bacon, green pepper — the possibilities are endless. Serve your pizza with a salad.

Tips

If you make the crust with pumpkin (see variation) and omit the cheese, you can enjoy pizza from stage 4 of the intro diet.

Make sure to prepare the beans properly, as described on page 72. Keep in mind that, even after this preparation, some people may find them difficult or impossible to digest.

Sesame flour is available online and at some well-stocked health food stores.

- **Preheat oven to 425°F (220°C), with rack set in second-lowest position**
- **Nut grinder (see box, page 75)**
- **Blender**
- **Baking sheet, greased or lined with parchment paper**

Pizza Dough

5 oz	dried soaked hazelnuts (see page 74)	150 g
3½ oz	cooked white beans (see page 72)	100 g
¼ cup	sesame flour	60 mL
1 tsp	dried oregano	5 mL
½ tsp	salt	2 mL
1	large egg, beaten	1
1 tbsp	unflavored gelatin powder	15 mL

Tomato Sauce

2 tbsp	cooking fat	30 mL
1	small onion, finely chopped	1
½	stalk celery, finely chopped	½
2	cloves garlic, minced	2
½ tsp	dried thyme	2 mL
⅔ cup	crushed tomatoes (from a jar)	150 mL
6 tbsp	water	90 mL
1 tsp	tomato vinegar	5 mL

Toppings

	Cooking fat	
7 oz	ground beef, veal or lamb	200 g
	Freshly ground black pepper	
10	mushrooms, sliced	10
⅔ cup	shredded Swiss cheese	150 mL
	Dried oregano	

1. *Dough:* In nut grinder, grind hazelnuts into medium-fine flour.

2. In blender, process beans, hazelnut flour, sesame flour, oregano and salt until smooth. Transfer to a bowl.

3. Add egg to bean mixture and knead until dough comes together.

Tips

Choose a good-quality brand of unflavored gelatin powder made from grass-fed animals, such as Great Lakes or Vital Protein. For more information, see page 55.

Tomato vinegar can be purchased online. It adds a wonderful umami flavor, but if you don't have it on hand, you can substitute a good-quality no-sugar-added balsamic vinegar.

Variation

The cooked white beans will yield a firm dough and a crispy crust, but if you cannot tolerate them, you can use 5 oz (150 g) Baked Pumpkin or Squash (page 77) or cooked cauliflower, which will yield a more liquid dough and a decent crust.

4. On prepared baking sheet, form dough into a large circle, about 12 inches (30 cm) in diameter, pressing and spreading it to make it as thin as possible without it crumbling.

5. Sprinkle gelatin over dough in an even layer and gently press into dough.

6. Bake in preheated oven for 15 minutes. Remove crust from oven and set aside. Position oven rack in middle of oven and increase temperature to 435°F (225°C).

7. *Sauce:* In a small saucepan, heat cooking fat over medium heat. Add onion and celery; cook, stirring, for about 2 minutes or until translucent. Add garlic and thyme; cook, stirring, for 30 seconds. Stir in tomatoes and water. Reduce heat and simmer, stirring occasionally, for 15 to 20 minutes or until slightly thickened.

8. Transfer sauce to blender, add tomato vinegar and process until smooth. Set aside.

9. *Toppings:* In a skillet, melt a thin layer of cooking fat over medium-high heat. Add ground meat and season with pepper; cook, stirring and breaking meat up, for about 8 minutes or until browned and no longer pink. Remove from heat.

10. Spread tomato sauce on baked crust. Spread meat over sauce, top with mushrooms and sprinkle with cheese.

11. Bake pizza on middle rack for about 10 minutes or until toppings are hot and cheese is melted. Sprinkle oregano on top.

Variation

If you want to spice up the flavor, make a tapenade to spread over the prebaked crust in step 10, before adding the tomato sauce. To make tapenade, mash 10 pitted olives (pit them yourself; they taste so much better than the store-bought pitted ones), 2 anchovies, 2 cloves of garlic and 2 crushed small dried chile peppers into a paste.

Corned Tongue in Mushroom Sauce

Here's yet another old-fashioned recipe! This was my absolute favorite dish when I was growing up. During the long cooking time, the tongue becomes extremely soft and tasty! Set aside 24 to 48 hours to corn the tongue before cooking the dish. Mashed Root Vegetables (page 181) and Creamed Celery Root (page 175) pair well with corned tongue. When you're transitioning out of the GAPS diet, it's also excellent with mashed potatoes with lots of butter.

Tip

When tongue is fully cooked, it can be easily peeled. If you feel resistance, it hasn't cooked long enough; return it to the pot and simmer longer.

• *Blender*

Corning Brine

4 cups	water	1 L
8 oz	salt	250 g
1 tbsp	honey	15 mL
	Small handful whole black peppercorns	
	Small handful whole coriander seeds	
	Small handful mustard seeds	
4 or 5	bay leaves	4 or 5
12 cups	cold water	3 L
1	calf's tongue (1 to 2 lbs/500 g) or beef tongue (up to 4 lbs/2 kg)	1
16 cups	water (or enough to cover the tongue)	4 L
1	onion	1
1	large carrot	1
1	thick slice celery root	1
1 tsp	salt (approx.)	5 mL
	Small handful whole black peppercorns	
1/4 cup	butter	60 mL
1 lb	mushrooms, halved	500 g
	Chopped fresh parsley	

1. *Corning Brine:* In a large pot, combine 4 cups (1 L) water, salt, honey, peppercorns, coriander seeds, mustard seeds and bay leaves; bring to a boil over high heat, stirring to dissolve salt. Remove from heat and stir in cold water. Let cool completely.

2. Transfer brine to a nonreactive container, place tongue in brine, cover and refrigerate for 24 to 48 hours.

3. Discard brine and rinse tongue in fresh cold water. Place tongue in a clean pot and add water to cover. Add onion, carrot, celery root, salt and peppercorns; bring to a simmer over medium heat. Reduce heat to low, cover and simmer for 1 1/2 hours for a calf's tongue or up to 3 hours for a beef tongue, or until tender (see tip).

Tips
You can remove the pepper-corns from the sauce or leave them in, as you prefer.

You will have a lot of sauce. You can serve it all as is or reduce it by letting it cook uncovered for a while. Or reserve some to add to your daily bone broth!

4. Remove tongue from pot and let cool slightly. Peel off outer layer. Carve tongue crosswise into $\frac{1}{4}$-inch (0.5 cm) slices.

5. Using a slotted spoon, transfer onion, carrot and celery root to blender, along with a little cooking liquid; blend until mashed, then return to the pot.

6. In a large skillet, melt butter over medium-high heat. Add mushrooms and cook, stirring, for about 6 minutes or until tender and lightly browned.

7. Add mushrooms to sauce, along with tongue slices; simmer until heated through. Taste and adjust seasoning with salt.

8. Serve with a bowl of parsley to sprinkle on top.

Variation
Substitute asparagus for the mushrooms and replace the parsley with dill, or just sprinkle the tongue with green olive slices.

Osso Buco

Also known as osso buco Milanese, this classic recipe needs no alteration to be GAPS-friendly. It is ideally designed to provide good taste, satisfaction and nourishment. "Osso buco" refers to the hole in the bones, where the marrow is, and boy, do we want this! The gremolata garnish only enhances the heavenly flavor. Serve Mashed Root Vegetables (page 181) alongside.

Tips

Don't forget to eat the bone marrow too!

Reserve and freeze leftover bones and cartilage to make Bone Broth (page 99).

Tomato vinegar can be purchased online. It adds a wonderful umami flavor, but if you don't have it on hand, you can substitute a good-quality no-sugar-added balsamic vinegar.

4	slices bone-in veal shank (about 2½ lbs/1.25 kg total)	4
	Salt	
	Animal fat or Clarified Butter (page 68)	
3	stalks celery, sliced	3
2	onions, sliced	2
4	cloves garlic, minced	4
¾ cup	tomato purée	175 mL
½ cup	dry white or red wine	125 mL
1 tbsp	tomato vinegar	15 mL
	Freshly ground black pepper	

Gremolata

2	handfuls fresh parsley, finely chopped	2
2	cloves garlic, minced	2
	Grated zest of 1 lemon	

1. Sprinkle veal slices on both sides with a little salt. In a large, wide pot, melt ¼ cup (60 mL) cooking fat over high heat. Add veal and brown on both sides. Transfer to a plate.

2. Reduce heat to medium-low and add more fat to the pot, if necessary. Add celery and onions; cook, stirring, for about 4 minutes or until translucent. Add garlic and cook, stirring, for 30 seconds.

3. Stir in tomato purée, wine and tomato vinegar. Grind pepper into the sauce and return veal and any accumulated juices to pot, turning veal to coat. Reduce heat to low, cover and simmer for about 1 hour or until meat is very tender and falling off the bone.

4. *Gremolata:* In a bowl, combine parsley, garlic and lemon zest.

5. Serve meat in sauce with a bowl of gremolata to sprinkle on top.

Veal Tails in Red Wine

This ragoût needs to simmer for quite some time, but it's a real treat when you have time for it. It is very GAPS-friendly because of the high gelatin content in the bones. Serve it with Mashed Root Vegetables (page 181), Oven-Baked Vegetables (page 180), Carrot and Zucchini Spaghetti (page 182) or Cauliflower Couscous (page 174).

Tips

Veal tails may be difficult to find, so be sure to call ahead to a butcher or large supermarket to order them in advance. Oxtails may be substituted for the veal tails.

Reserve leftover bones to make more bone broth. They are loaded with gelatin.

	Clarified Butter (page 68) or other animal fat	
2 lbs	veal tails, cut into pieces	1 kg
3	carrots, cut into 1¼-inch (3 cm) pieces	3
2	onions, cut into quarters	2
1	stalk celery, cut into 1¼-inch (3 cm) pieces	1
	Salt and freshly ground black pepper	
1 tsp	dried thyme (or 2 fresh sprigs)	5 mL
1	bay leaf	1
¾ cup	Bone Broth (page 99)	175 mL
½ cup	dry red wine	125 mL
½ to 1 cup	water	125 to 250 mL

1. In a pot, melt ¼ cup (60 mL) cooking fat over high heat. Add veal pieces, in batches as necessary, and brown on all sides. Transfer to a bowl.

2. Reduce heat to medium-low and add a little more fat to the pot. Add carrots, onions and celery; cook, stirring, for about 4 minutes or until onions are translucent.

3. Return veal and any accumulated juices to the pot. Season with salt and pepper and add thyme and bay leaf. Stir in broth and wine. Reduce heat to low, cover and simmer for 3 hours, adding water as necessary, until meat is very tender and falling off the bones. Discard bay leaf. Taste and adjust seasoning with salt and pepper.

Veal Heart Casserole

Organ meat may be considered old-fashioned, and you might have to order it from your butcher in advance, but it's loaded with nutrition and flavor! This tasty casserole goes well with Cauliflower Couscous (page 174), Oven-Baked Vegetables (page 180) or Mashed Root Vegetables (page 181).

Tips

Purchase bacon that is free of additives aside from salt.

Tomato vinegar can be purchased online. It adds a wonderful umami flavor, but if you don't have it on hand, you can substitute a good-quality no-sugar-added balsamic vinegar.

Reserve and freeze the cut-away parts from step 1 for future bone broth preparation.

Use plenty of cooking fat, as heart meat is lean.

14 oz	veal or beef heart	400 g
	Salt	
	Animal fat	
2 oz	bacon (see tip), finely chopped	60 g
3	carrots, sliced	3
2	large onions, sliced	2
1	stalk celery, sliced	1
1 tsp	dried rosemary	5 mL
1⅔ cups	crushed tomatoes (from a jar)	400 mL
1 cup	Bone Broth (page 99)	250 mL
	Freshly ground black pepper	
1 tbsp	tomato vinegar	15 mL

1. Remove sinew, veins and fat from heart (see tip). Rinse heart in cold water, pat dry and cut into bite-size pieces. Sprinkle with salt.

2. In a large pot, melt plenty of animal fat over high heat. Add heart pieces, in batches as necessary, and brown on all sides. Transfer to a plate.

3. Add bacon to the pot and cook, stirring, until crisp. Reduce heat to medium-low, add more animal fat as necessary, then add carrots, onions and celery; cook, stirring, for 4 to 5 minutes or until onions are translucent.

4. Stir in rosemary, tomatoes and broth, then stir in heart pieces and any accumulated juices. Season with pepper. Reduce heat to low, cover and simmer, stirring occasionally, for about 25 minutes or until heart is tender. Stir in tomato vinegar. Taste and adjust seasoning with salt and pepper.

Lamb Meatballs in Spicy Tomato Sauce

Makes 4 servings

A spicy tomato sauce really livens up lamb meatballs. Serve them with the delicious vegetables of your choice.

Tips

Use between 2 and 4 tbsp (30 and 60 mL) cooking fat in step 1, depending on your preference and how much fat you need in your diet.

You can use any other kind of ground meat, and can adjust the amounts of the spices to your taste.

If you prefer, you can form the meat mixture into oblong koftas instead of meatballs.

Tomato Sauce

	Cooking fat	
1	large onion, finely chopped	1
1	slice celery root, finely chopped	1
2	cloves garlic, minced	2
1 tsp	garam masala	5 mL
1/2 tsp	ground cardamom	2 mL
Pinch	cayenne pepper	Pinch
1²/₃ cups	crushed tomatoes (from a jar)	400 mL
²/₃ cup	Bone Broth (page 99)	150 mL
	Salt and freshly ground black pepper	

Lamb Meatballs

	ground lamb	500 g
1 lb	ground lamb	500 g
2	cloves garlic, minced	2
	Juice of 1/2 lemon	
	Salt and freshly ground black pepper	
	Cooking fat	

1. *Tomato Sauce:* In a saucepan, heat desired amount of cooking fat (see tip) over medium heat. Add onion and celery root; cook, stirring, for 5 minutes or until softened. Stir in garlic, garam masala, cardamom and cayenne; cook, stirring, for 30 seconds.

2. Stir in crushed tomatoes and broth. Season to taste with salt and pepper. Reduce heat to low, cover and simmer for about 20 minutes or until flavors are blended.

3. *Lamb Meatballs:* In a bowl, combine lamb, garlic, lemon juice, salt and pepper. Form into 16 meatballs.

4. In a large skillet, heat 2 tbsp (30 mL) cooking fat over medium-high heat. Add meatballs, in batches as necessary, reduce heat to medium-low and fry, turning once, for about 5 minutes per side or until no longer pink inside and a meat thermometer inserted in the thickest part of a meatball registers 160°F (71°C). Pour tomato sauce over meatballs.

Lamb-Stuffed Spinach Pancakes

Makes 4 servings

It takes a while to prepare this dish, but you can team up with helpful kids or friends and have fun with it. The result is appreciated by gourmets of all ages. Serve the stuffed pancakes with a fresh green salad.

Tip

If the cooking temperature is too low in step 1, the meat will boil instead of frying.

- **Preheat oven to 400°F (200°C), with rack set in second-lowest position**
- **13- by 9-inch (33 by 23 cm) lasagna dish, greased**

	Animal fat, butter or Clarified Butter (page 68)	
14 oz	ground lamb	400 g
1	small onion, finely chopped	1
1	large carrot, finely diced	1
½ tsp	ground allspice	2 mL
½ tsp	ground cinnamon	2 mL
¼ tsp	ground cloves	1 mL
Pinch	cayenne pepper	Pinch
1 tsp	salt	5 mL
	Freshly ground black pepper	
4	cloves garlic, minced	4
1¼ cups	crushed tomatoes (from a jar)	300 mL
¾ cup	Bone Broth (page 99)	175 mL
4	Spinach Pancakes (page 118)	4
⅔ cup	shredded Swiss cheese	75 g

1. In a pot, melt cooking fat over medium-high heat. Add half the lamb and cook, stirring and breaking it up, until no longer pink. Transfer to a plate. Repeat with the remaining lamb, adding more fat and adjusting heat between batches as necessary.

2. Reduce heat to medium-low and add more fat to the pot, if necessary. Add onion, carrot, allspice, cinnamon, cloves, cayenne, salt and pepper to taste; cook, stirring, for about 3 minutes or until onion is translucent. Add garlic and cook, stirring, for 30 seconds.

3. Return meat and any accumulated juices to the pot. Stir in crushed tomatoes and broth. Reduce heat to low, cover and simmer while you make the pancakes.

4. Make 4 spinach pancakes, following the directions on page 118.

5. Taste meat filling and adjust spices, if desired.

6. Place 1 pancake in prepared dish. Place one-quarter of the meat filling in a wide strip crosswise, roll up pancake and turn seam side down. Repeat with remaining pancakes and filling, then arrange pancakes in dish with sides touching. Sprinkle with cheese.

7. Bake in preheated oven for 25 minutes or until filling is hot and cheese is melted.

Spicy Apple Compote

Makes about 3 cups (750 mL)

Apples are fantastic because they work well with both sweet and salty dishes. This compote can be served as a side dish with fatty fish, like mackerel or salmon, or with meats such as pork and lamb.

Tips

Cooking apples that soften when cooked, such as McIntosh, Ida Red, Golden Delicious and Empire, are best for this recipe.

Adjust the amount of chile peppers according to your taste and heat tolerance.

Store compote in a glass jar in the refrigerator for up to 5 days.

• *Juicer*

1½ lbs	cooking apples (about 6 to 8 small)	750 g
	Water	
2 tbsp	coconut oil	30 mL
2 tsp	grated gingerroot	10 mL
1 tsp	curry powder	5 mL
1	onion, grated	1
1	stalk celery, thinly sliced	1
½	red bell pepper, thinly sliced	½
2	cloves garlic, minced	2
2	small fresh or dried whole chile peppers (or ¼ tsp/1 mL chili powder)	2
1 tsp	whole black peppercorns	5 mL
1 tsp	salt	5 mL

1. Peel apples, if desired. Quarter apples and trim out cores, reserving cores; cut each quarter in half.

2. In juicer, process apple cores. Measure the amount of juice and add enough water to make 6 tbsp (90 mL) liquid.

3. In a pot, heat coconut oil over high heat. Add ginger and curry powder; cook, stirring, for 1 minute. Reduce heat to medium-low. Add onion, celery and red pepper; cook, stirring, for about 2 minutes or until translucent.

4. Stir in apple pieces, garlic, chiles, peppercorns, salt and apple juice; cover and simmer, stirring occasionally, for about 30 minutes or until apples are softened and compote is thickened. Remove and discard chiles (leave peppercorns in the compote).

White Asparagus with Lemon Butter

Makes 4 servings

Asparagus has been prepared all over the world in many ways for thousands of years. This simple preparation really helps the delicate taste unfold.

Tips

White asparagus is available for only a short time each year and is just too delicious to overlook. But if you cannot find it, you can also use green asparagus. Double up the amount per person and cook the spears for 4 to 8 minutes, depending on thickness.

If you don't plan to cook white asparagus immediately after peeling it, place it in a bowl of cold water acidified with lemon juice.

If you happen to have an asparagus pot, use it! Because this specialized pot is tall and narrow, the stalks cook in the water while the tender heads just get steamed.

This dish can also be served as an appetizer. Allow 2 to 4 asparagus spears per person.

8 to 16	spears white asparagus (see tip)	8 to 16
6 tbsp + 2 tsp	butter or Clarified Butter (page 68)	100 mL
1/2 tsp	freshly squeezed lemon juice	2 mL

1. Peel asparagus stalks. The bottom part often has the woodiest peel, so it should be peeled with great care. The tips need only be rinsed.

2. In a pot or large skillet of simmering lightly salted water, cook asparagus for 9 to 15 minutes, depending on thickness. To test for doneness, insert the tip of a sharp knife into the thickest stalk to check if it is the desired tenderness. If their thickness varies greatly, you may remove the spears one by one as they are done.

3. In a small saucepan, melt butter over low heat. Stir in lemon juice.

4. Drain asparagus and immediately wrap in a clean tea towel to soak up excess water and keep asparagus warm. Arrange on a platter and drizzle with lemon butter.

Variations

If you omit the lemon juice, asparagus is fine from stage 3 of the intro diet.

Asparagus is also good with Béarnaise Sauce (page 186) in place of the lemon butter.

Sweet-and-Sour Red Cabbage

Makes 8 servings

Sweet and sour flavors really highlight the fine taste of red cabbage. For us Gapsters, that's where dates and apple cider vinegar come in handy. This dish is the perfect accompaniment to roast pork, duck or meatballs. Served cold, it complements veal or duck liver pâté.

Tips

Use between 4 and 6 tbsp (60 and 90 mL) cooking fat in step 2, depending on your preference and how much fat you need in your diet.

You can make this dish ahead of time and store it in clean mason jars in the refrigerator for up to 2 weeks.

1	head red cabbage (about 2 lbs/1 kg)	1
	Duck fat, goose fat or lard	
15	dates, pitted and diced	15
1 cup	unsweetened apple cider (approx.)	250 mL
3 tbsp	apple cider vinegar (approx.)	45 mL
1 to 1½ tsp	salt	5 to 7 mL

1. Remove outer leaves from cabbage head and cut out core. Shred cabbage.

2. In a large pot, melt a generous amount of cooking fat (see tip) over medium heat. Add cabbage and cook, stirring, for about 5 minutes or until starting to wilt.

3. Stir in dates, cider, vinegar and 1 tsp (5 mL) salt; reduce heat to low, cover and simmer for 30 to 45 minutes or until cabbage is desired doneness. Taste and adjust seasoning as desired with salt, vinegar and/or cider.

Cauliflower Gratin

Makes 3 to
4 servings

*This gratin is enriched
with lentils and almonds,
making it a meal in its own
right if you're in the mood
for a vegetarian dinner.
Serve your favorite salad
alongside.*

Tip

Make sure to prepare the
lentils properly, as described
on page 73. Keep in
mind that, even after this
preparation, some people
may find them difficult or
impossible to digest.

- *Preheat oven to 375°F (190°C), with rack set in second-lowest position*
- *8-cup (2 L) gratin dish, greased with butter or Clarified Butter (page 68)*
- *Nut grinder (see box, page 75)*
- *Electric mixer*

1	head cauliflower, cut into quarters	1
1 oz	dried soaked almonds (see page 74)	30 g
3	large eggs, separated	3
½ cup	cooked red lentils (see page 73)	125 mL
Pinch	grated nutmeg	Pinch
	Salt and freshly ground black pepper	
2 tbsp	butter or Clarified Butter (page 68)	30 mL

1. In a pot of boiling lightly salted water, blanch cauliflower for 3 minutes. Drain and rinse under cold water to stop the cooking. Drain well, then place in prepared gratin dish.

2. In nut grinder, grind almonds to the consistency of bread crumbs.

3. In a bowl, whisk together egg yolks, lentils and nutmeg. Season with salt and pepper.

4. In another bowl, using the electric mixer, beat egg whites until stiff. Using a silicone spatula, carefully fold egg whites into lentil mixture.

5. Spread lentil mixture evenly over cauliflower, sprinkle with almond crumbs and distribute thin slices of butter on top.

6. Bake in preheated oven for 30 minutes or until top is golden.

Cauliflower Couscous

Makes 4 servings

Often used as a starch in North African cuisine, couscous is really a wheat product consisting of tiny, round yellowish grains. It is too starchy for Gapsters, so here is an alternative you can serve as part of a buffet, as a lunch salad or as an accompaniment for stews and casseroles.

Tips

You can prepare the dish through step 3, cover and refrigerate for up to 1 day before proceeding with step 4.

If you're serving this dish as part of a buffet dinner, it makes 8 servings.

In step 2, start the timer when the water returns to a boil.

- *High-speed blender or food processor*

½	large head cauliflower (or 1 small), about 1 lb (500 g)	½
¼ cup	cold-pressed olive oil	60 mL
1 tbsp	raw honey	15 mL
	Juice of 1 lime	
1	small clove garlic, minced	1
Pinch	cayenne pepper	Pinch
	Salt and freshly ground black pepper	
2½ oz	dried soaked almonds (see page 74), chopped	75 g
1 tbsp	flax seeds	15 mL
1 tbsp	sesame seeds	15 mL
2	large tomatoes, chopped, divided	2
1	bunch fresh cilantro, parsley or other herbs, chopped, divided	1

1. Cut cauliflower into small pieces and process in blender to the consistency of couscous. This happens quickly! Be sure not to purée it.

2. Add cauliflower to a pot of boiling lightly salted water, cover and blanch for 30 to 60 seconds or until al dente. Drain and rinse cauliflower under cold running water to stop the cooking. Drain well.

3. In a large bowl, whisk together olive oil, honey, lime juice, garlic, cayenne, and salt and pepper to taste. Add cauliflower, almonds, flax seeds, sesame seeds, half the tomatoes and half the cilantro, stirring gently to coat.

4. Transfer to a serving bowl and garnish with remaining tomatoes and cilantro.

Creamed Celery Root

Makes 2 to 4 servings

This extremely easy side dish can be served warm or cold, and it goes well with fish, meat, poultry or any supper pie. Try it with Spinach Pie (page 178)!

Tip
Chop only the parsley leaves and reserve the stems for making Bone Broth (page 99) or for juicing.

	Clarified Butter (page 68)	
1	small celery root (or ½ large), diced	1
	Salt and freshly ground black pepper	
2 tbsp	Sour Cream (page 92)	30 mL
	Chopped fresh parsley	

1. In a skillet, melt desired amount of clarified butter over medium-low heat. Stir in celery root and season to taste with salt and pepper. Reduce heat to low, cover and simmer, stirring occasionally, for 20 to 30 minutes or until tender.

2. Stir in sour cream and sprinkle with parsley.

Leeks au Gratin

Makes 4 servings

This dish turns leeks into the star of the meal!

- **Preheat oven to 375°F (190°C), with rack set in second-lowest position**
- **8-inch (20 cm) square shallow baking dish**

4	leeks (white and light green parts only)	4
2½ tbsp	butter or Clarified Butter (page 68), melted	37 mL
⅔ cup	shredded Swiss cheese	150 mL
½ tsp	lightly crushed pink peppercorns	2 mL

1. Cut leeks in half lengthwise, rinse thoroughly and pat dry.

2. Brush baking dish with a thin coating of melted butter. Arrange leeks, cut side up, in a single layer in dish. Drizzle evenly with the remaining butter. Sprinkle cheese and peppercorns evenly over top.

3. Bake in preheated oven for about 25 minutes or until leeks are tender and soft.

Stuffed Portobello Mushrooms

Makes 4 servings

These mushrooms are nice for lunch, as a starter, as a side dish, on a buffet or as an alternative to processed snacks.

Tips

Other varieties of mushrooms can be used if they are about 2 to 3 inches (5 to 7.5 cm) in diameter so that they form a small bowl once the stems are removed and the caps are turned upside down.

Use between 2 and 4 tbsp (30 and 60 mL) cooking fat in step 2, depending on your preference and how much fat you need in your diet.

- *Preheat oven to 350°F (180°C), with rack set in middle position*
- *Large shallow baking dish, greased*

8	portobello mushrooms (2 to 3 inches/5 to 7.5 cm in diameter)	8
	Butter	
2 to 3	small shallots, minced	2 to 3
2	cloves garlic, minced	2
3 tbsp	chopped fresh parsley	45 mL
	Salt and freshly ground black pepper	
½ cup	shredded Swiss cheese	125 mL

1. Trim stems from mushrooms caps; set caps aside and chop stems.

2. In a small skillet, melt desired amount of butter (see tip) over medium-low heat. Add mushroom stems, shallots to taste, garlic, parsley, salt to taste and plenty of pepper; cook, stirring, for 5 minutes or until tender. Remove from heat.

3. Place mushroom caps, smooth side down, in prepared baking dish. Spoon shallot mixture into caps and sprinkle with cheese.

4. Bake in preheated oven for 15 minutes or until mushrooms are tender and cheese is melted.

Mushrooms with Spinach

Makes 4 servings

A small amount of healing bone broth adds even more delicious flavor to this spicy vegetable dish.

1 tbsp	cooking fat	15 mL
1	small onion, coarsely chopped	1
1 tsp	ground turmeric	5 mL
1/2 tsp	ground coriander	2 mL
1/4 tsp	cayenne pepper	1 mL
8 oz	mushrooms, cut in half	250 g
1 lb	frozen spinach, thawed, squeezed dry and coarsely chopped	500 g
1/4 cup	Bone Broth (page 99)	60 mL
	Salt and freshly ground black pepper	

1. In a skillet, heat cooking fat over low heat. Stir in onion, turmeric, coriander and cayenne. Cover and cook for 5 to 10 minutes or until tender.

2. Add mushrooms and cook, stirring occasionally, for about 2 minutes or until starting to soften.

3. Add spinach and bone broth, stirring well. Cover and simmer for 15 minutes. Season to taste with salt and pepper.

Variations

If you substitute Chicken or Veal Stock (page 102) for the bone broth, you can enjoy this recipe from stage 5 of the intro diet.

To turn this into a lunch dish reminiscent of spinach Florentine, make 4 indentations in the vegetable mixture in the pan at the end of step 3 and crack an egg into each. Cover and simmer until the egg whites are set. Sprinkle with chopped fresh parsley.

Spinach Pie

Makes 6 servings

How do you make a crisp crust when you cannot use flour? Here's one possibility. Bring a pie (or 6 smaller ones) along on your next picnic, serve some for lunch or enjoy some with a nice salad for dinner. The pie is also easy to freeze and thaw quickly, in case you have unexpected guests.

Tip

Choose a good-quality brand of unflavored gelatin powder made from grass-fed animals, such as Great Lakes or Vital Protein. For more information, see page 55.

- *Preheat oven to 350°F (180°C), with rack set in second-lowest position*
- *Nut grinder (see box, page 75)*
- *Blender*
- *9-inch (23 cm) pie plate, greased*

Crust

7 oz	dried soaked nuts (see page 74), divided	200 g
2 tbsp	butter or Clarified Butter (page 68)	30 mL
1 cup	cooked white beans or lima beans (see page 72)	250 mL
½ tsp	salt	2 mL
2	large eggs	2
2 tsp	unflavored gelatin powder	10 mL

Filling

1 lb	frozen whole spinach, thawed	500 g
3 tbsp	cooking fat	45 mL
1 tsp	ground turmeric	5 mL
½ tsp	ground coriander	2 mL
Pinch	cayenne pepper	Pinch
1 to 2	cloves garlic, minced	1 to 2
1	large carrot, coarsely grated	1
1	small onion, chopped	1
2	large eggs	2
1 tbsp	Sour Cream (page 92)	15 mL
¼ to ½ tsp	salt	1 to 2 mL
¼ to ½ tsp	freshly ground black pepper	1 to 2 mL
6 tbsp	shredded cheese (such as Swiss)	90 mL

1. *Crust:* In nut grinder, grind half the nuts into fine flour and transfer to a bowl. Grind the remaining nuts into medium-fine flour and add to fine flour.

2. Using a pastry blender, two knives or your fingers, crumble butter into nut flours to achieve the consistency of grated cheese.

3. In blender, process nut flour mixture, beans, salt and eggs until smooth.

Make sure to prepare the beans properly, as described on page 72. Keep in mind that, even after this preparation, some people may find them difficult or impossible to digest.

4. Spread dough in prepared pie plate, in a thin, even layer, making sure to cover the edges of the plate. Trim off any excess dough from the edges. Sprinkle gelatin over crust in a thin layer and gently press into dough.

5. Bake crust in preheated oven for 25 minutes or until golden (it will firm up when cooled).

6. *Filling:* Meanwhile, squeeze excess water from thawed spinach, coarsely chop it and gently pat it dry.

7. In a skillet, melt cooking fat over medium heat. Stir in turmeric, coriander and cayenne, then stir in spinach, garlic to taste, carrot and onion. Cover and cook for 5 minutes or until tender. Remove from heat.

8. In a bowl, whisk eggs until blended. Stir into skillet, along with sour cream. Season with salt and pepper.

9. Pour filling into prebaked crust and sprinkle with cheese.

10. Bake pie for 20 minutes or until filling is set. Let cool for 10 minutes. Serve warm or let cool to room temperature.

Variation

Instead of making one big pie, you can make 6 individual pies, each about 3 inches (7.5 cm) in diameter. Prebake the crusts for 15 minutes and bake the filled pies for about 12 minutes or until filling is set.

Oven-Baked Vegetables

Makes 4 servings

This recipe is really just a launching pad for your creativity, as you can use any GAPS-friendly vegetables you please. Whatever you choose, it will make a good accompaniment to fish, poultry and meat.

Tip

Make sure to prepare the beans properly, as described on page 72. Keep in mind that, even after this preparation, some people may find them difficult or impossible to digest.

- *Preheat oven to 350°F (180°C)*
- *8-cup (2 L) shallow baking dish*

¼ cup	butter, Clarified Butter (page 68) or animal fat	60 mL
6	large carrots, cut into large chunks	6
2	large leeks (white and light green parts only), cut into large chunks	2
4	tomatoes, quartered	4
2 cups	cubed Hokkaido, Red Kuri or other winter squash (1-inch/2.5 cm cubes)	500 mL
1¼ cups	cooked white beans (see page 72)	300 mL
	Fresh thyme sprigs	
	Salt	

1. Generously coat baking dish with cooking fat.

2. In a large pot of boiling water, boil carrots and leeks for 5 minutes. Drain, pat dry and place in prepared baking dish.

3. Add tomatoes, squash and beans, stirring well to make sure everything is covered with cooking fat. Add thyme and sprinkle with salt.

4. Bake in preheated oven for 30 minutes or until vegetables are tender.

Variations

Add shredded Swiss cheese to the vegetables before adding the thyme and salt.

If you omit the beans, you can enjoy this dish from stage 4 of the intro diet.

Mashed Root Vegetables

| Makes 4 servings | | |

Before you start following the GAPS diet, you might expect that you will miss starchy foods like potatoes, rice and pasta. The solution is to make great alternatives! This mash provides flavor, nourishment and texture as a side dish to casseroles, roasts and more.

Tips

Save the cooking water to make stock (page 102), bone broth (page 99) or soup, or drink it for a nutrient boost.

Use leftovers to make Root Vegetable Patties (page 136) to add to a lunch bag.

- **Immersion blender**

5 oz	beets, sliced	150 g
12 oz	carrots, sliced or cut into chunks	375 g
14 oz	celery root, sliced or cut into chunks	400 g
6 tbsp	Clarified Butter (page 68)	90 mL
	Grated nutmeg	
	Salt and freshly ground black pepper	
	Chopped fresh parsley	

1. Add beets to a medium saucepan of boiling lightly salted water. Reduce heat to medium and cook for 30 minutes.

2. Add carrots and celery root; cook for 30 minutes or until vegetables are very tender. Drain vegetables (see tip) and return to the pot.

3. Add butter to the pot and, using the immersion blender, purée root vegetables until smooth. Season to taste with nutmeg, salt and pepper.

4. Serve with a bowl of parsley to sprinkle over top.

Variations

Other vegetable options include broccoli, cauliflower and pumpkin. Adjust the cooking times as needed for very tender vegetables.

If you tolerate cooked white beans (page 72), blend them into the purée in step 3.

Add raw crushed garlic to the purée with the nutmeg.

Carrot and Zucchini Spaghetti

Makes 4 servings

Regular pasta is difficult for Gapsters to digest, so here's an excellent alternative. Spiralizers are easy to find in kitchen stores these days and make the task even quicker (and more fun). Serve these "noodles" just as you would your usual spaghetti!

Tips

You may, of course, also use other GAPS-friendly vegetables, such as celery.

If using a vegetable peeler, when the vegetables become so thin you can't hold them, place them on a cutting board and use a sharp knife to cut as many strips as possible. Cook any leftover pieces to serve for lunch the next day, or store them in the refrigerator for your next batch of juice.

- **Vegetable peeler or spiralizer**

2 lbs	carrots	1 kg
2	zucchini or yellow summer squash	2
8 cups	water	2 L
1 tsp	salt	5 mL
	Cold-pressed olive oil	

1. Using the peeler, shred carrots and zucchini.

2. In a pot, bring water and salt to a boil over high heat. Add carrot and zucchini strips, reduce heat and simmer for about 3 minutes or until tender. (Use a fork to fish out a strip and check if it is done.)

3. Drain vegetables (see tip, page 181) well in a colander before returning them to the pot. Drizzle a little olive oil on top before serving.

Mushroom Fish Sauce

| Makes 3 to 4 servings |

This sauce is a really good way to spice up a simple fish dish. Just steam fish in butter (or any other cooking fat), season it with salt and pepper, serve it with this sauce and add well-cooked vegetables or a fresh salad on the side, and you have a perfect meal!

Tips

Use between 2 and 4 tbsp (30 and 60 mL) cooking fat in step 1, depending on your preference and how much fat you need in your diet.

In step 2, simmer covered or uncovered, depending on how much you want to reduce the stock.

	Butter or Clarified Butter (page 68)	
1	stalk celery, chopped	1
½	onion, chopped	½
8 oz	mushrooms, halved	250 g
¾ cup	Fish Stock (page 103) or Fish Bone Broth (page 101)	175 mL
	Salt and freshly ground black pepper	

1. In a saucepan, melt desired amount of butter (see tip) over medium heat. Stir in celery and onion; cover and cook for about 15 minutes or until translucent. Stir in mushrooms, cover and cook for 5 minutes or until tender.

2. Add stock and simmer for 5 minutes (see tip). Season to taste with salt and pepper.

Gravlax Sauce

**Makes about
¼ cup (60 mL)**

*This sauce is a heavenly
match for Gravlax
(page 121), but is also
good with ham.*

Tips

Grind the fennel seeds using
a mortar and pestle or in a
spice grinder.

If using fresh dill, make
sure to rinse it and pat it dry
before use.

1 tsp	fennel seeds, freshly ground (see tip)	5 mL
2 tbsp	Dijon mustard	30 mL
2 tbsp	raw honey	30 mL
	Salt and freshly ground black pepper	
1 tbsp	chopped fresh dill (or 1 tsp/5 mL dried dillweed)	15 mL

1. In a small bowl, combine fennel, mustard and honey. Season to taste with salt and pepper, then stir in dill.

Horseradish Cream

**Makes about
6 tbsp (90 mL)**

*Coconut kefir is used to
make this spicy cream,
which reminds me of
wasabi. It's good with
GAPS Sushi (page 123)
and any cold meat, such
as a GAPS-friendly salami,
roast beef or cold tongue.*

⅓ cup	freshly grated horseradish	75 mL
5 tsp	Coconut Kefir (page 93)	25 mL

1. In a small bowl, combine horseradish and coconut kefir.

Peanut Butter Sauce

**Makes about
⅓ cup (75 mL)**

*This sauce goes well with
cooked or raw vegetables,
Thai dishes and chicken
(especially Chicken
Nuggets, page 131).*

Tips

In recipes that are not
heated, use raw honey for
its added health benefits.

If you prefer your sauce
a bit more fluid, you can
add more olive oil, but be
cautious with sesame oil,
as the flavor is potent!

• *Blender*

1	clove garlic, minced	1
2 tsp	grated gingerroot	10 mL
2 tbsp	natural peanut butter	30 mL
2 tbsp	cold-pressed olive oil	30 mL
1 tsp	cold-pressed sesame oil	5 mL
1 tsp	freshly squeezed lemon or lime juice	5 mL
½ tsp	raw honey	2 mL
Pinch	salt	Pinch

1. In blender, combine garlic, ginger, peanut butter, olive
   oil, sesame oil, lemon juice, honey and salt; blend until
   smooth. Taste and adjust seasoning as desired with salt
   and perhaps more garlic, ginger, lemon and/or honey.

Béarnaise Sauce

**Makes about
2 cups (500 mL)**

*Béarnaise sauce is very
GAPS-friendly, as it
contains clarified butter,
egg yolks and fresh parsley.
Serve it with hearty meats,
such as roast beef or steak.*

Tips

If you are lucky enough to
have a double boiler, now is
the time to use it!

Use only the clarified part of
the butter in step 4; discard
the white milky substance.
As with mayonnaise (see
step 2, page 187), add a very
small amount of butter at a
time to begin with, then add
gradually increasing amounts
while whisking continuously.

Make Béarnaise sauce as the
very last item on your dinner
menu, as it tends to cool fast
and curdle as it stands.

Essence

5 or 6	sprigs fresh parsley	5 or 6
1	small shallot, chopped	1
1	bay leaf	1
1 tsp	dried tarragon	5 mL
1/2 tsp	dried thyme	2 mL
	Small handful whole black peppercorns	
3 tbsp	white wine vinegar	45 mL
3 tbsp	dry white wine	45 mL

Sauce

1 1/4 cups	butter	300 mL
3	large egg yolks	3
2 tbsp	cold water	30 mL
	Salt and freshly ground black pepper	
	Dried tarragon	
	Chopped fresh parsley	
	Freshly squeezed lemon juice	

1. *Essence:* In a small saucepan, combine parsley, shallot, bay leaf, tarragon, thyme, peppercorns, vinegar and wine. Cover and bring to a simmer over medium-low heat. Simmer for about 15 minutes or until reduced by two-thirds. Strain out solids and let liquid cool completely.

2. *Sauce:* In a clean small saucepan, clarify butter over low heat (around 104°F/40°C) so that the oil rises and the white milky substance sinks to the bottom.

3. In a heatproof bowl set over a saucepan of simmering water (see tip), using an egg beater or handheld electric mixer, beat egg yolks, water and 2 tbsp (30 mL) essence until thick and airy. Keep an eye on the temperature of the simmering water. It should be held just at lukewarm; if it gets too hot, the sauce will coagulate. If the temperature rises too much (more than 104°F/40°C), just remove the bowl from the simmering water, returning it after a break so it doesn't get too cold either.

4. Still monitoring the temperature of the simmering water as above, gradually whisk clarified butter into egg mixture (see tip).

5. Season to taste with salt, pepper, tarragon, parsley and a little lemon juice. Serve immediately.

Mayonnaise

	Makes about ½ cup (125 mL)	
1	large egg yolk (see tip)	1
Pinch	salt	Pinch
1 tsp	Dijon mustard	5 mL
1 tsp	apple cider vinegar	5 mL
⅓ to ½ cup	cold-pressed olive oil	75 to 125 mL

Making your own mayonnaise allows you to use cold-pressed olive oil, which contains a lot of healing nutrients for body and mind. Mayonnaise serves as the base for several other cold sauces (see pages 188–189). Feel free to mix in a variety of herbs and spices and create your own custom version.

Tips

Publisher's note: Although raw eggs are considered nourishing in the GAPS diet, they may contain salmonella (see sidebar, page 22). If you prefer to err on the side of caution, use the yolk from a pasteurized in-shell egg, if they are available in your area. Note that, while pasteurized eggs are not part of the GAPS nutritional protocol, food safety must be your first priority.

If you add too much oil at a time, your mayonnaise may separate. If it does, you can: **a)** whisk the separated mayonnaise into a fresh egg yolk, starting with small drops; **b)** add a drop of cold water and beat vigorously in an effort to whisk it back together; **c)** refrigerate the bowl and beat again after a couple of hours.

1. In a small bowl, whisk egg yolk with salt until thickened. Whisk in mustard and vinegar.

2. Gradually pour in oil while whisking rapidly, starting with just a few drops at a time to keep mayonnaise from separating. Repeat the addition of a few drops of oil 12 to 20 times, then gradually increase the number of drops while whisking. When the first half of the oil has been whisked in, the remainder may be added in bigger drops. Continue adding oil until the mayonnaise is light, airy and emulsified.

3. Use immediately or cover tightly and store in the refrigerator for up to 2 days.

Aïoli

2	cloves garlic, crushed	2
Pinch	cayenne pepper	Pinch
½ cup	Mayonnaise (page 187)	125 mL

Makes about ½ cup (125 mL)

Aïoli is a good dip for raw vegetables or Sesame Crisps (page 199), but it also jazzes up fish soup or Fish Cakes (page 151).

1. In a small bowl, whisk garlic and cayenne into mayonnaise until well combined.

2. Use immediately or cover tightly and store in the refrigerator for up to 2 days.

Variation
If you omit the cayenne pepper, you can enjoy this recipe from stage 4 of the intro diet.

Green Sauce

⅓	small red onion, chopped	⅓
1 tbsp	drained capers, chopped	15 mL
½ cup	Mayonnaise (page 187)	125 mL
1	clove garlic, minced	1
	Small handful fresh dill, chopped	
3 tbsp	Sour Cream (page 92)	45 mL
1 tbsp	freshly squeezed lemon juice	15 mL
	Salt and freshly ground black pepper	

Makes about ½ cup (125 mL)

As long as you have homemade sour cream ready to go, this sauce is easy to prepare. It's good all year round with vegetables, fish and shellfish.

1. In a small bowl, fold red onion and capers into mayonnaise. Add garlic, dill, sour cream and lemon juice, stirring well. Season to taste with salt and pepper.

2. Use immediately or cover tightly and store in the refrigerator for up to 2 days.

Ravigote Sauce

**Makes about
2/3 cup (150 mL)**

*Ravigote sauce is good
with steamed carrots,
cauliflower, green peas
or green beans, and with
Fish Cakes (page 151) and
chicken (and potatoes
when you are transitioning
out of the GAPS diet).*

Tip

Chop only the parsley leaves
and reserve the stems for
making Bone Broth (page 99)
or for juicing.

	Handful fresh parsley, finely chopped	
1	small clove garlic, minced	1
1 tsp	minced drained capers	5 mL
1/4 tsp	dried tarragon	1 mL
	Freshly ground black pepper	
1/2 cup	Mayonnaise (page 187)	125 mL
1 1/2 tsp	apple cider vinegar	7 mL
1/2 tsp	Dijon mustard	2 mL
3 tbsp	Soft-Curd Cheese (page 71) or Sour Cream (page 92)	45 mL

1. In a small bowl, whisk together parsley, garlic, capers, tarragon, pepper to taste, mayonnaise, vinegar and mustard. Stir in soft-curd cheese.

2. Use immediately or cover tightly and store in the refrigerator for up to 2 days.

Rémoulade

**Makes about
2/3 cup (150 mL)**

*It may take a few extra
minutes to make your own
rémoulade, but the taste
is heavenly! It's the perfect
match for Fish Cakes
(page 151).*

Tips

To mash anchovies, push
them through a sieve.

If desired, you can add more
of any of the ingredients
to taste.

2	oil-packed anchovies, mashed	2
1	clove garlic, minced	1
	Handful fresh parsley, chopped	
2 tbsp	finely chopped drained sauerkraut	30 mL
1 tbsp	finely chopped drained capers	15 mL
1/4 tsp	dried tarragon	1 mL
1/2 cup	Mayonnaise (page 187)	125 mL
1 tsp	Dijon mustard	5 mL
	Salt and freshly ground black pepper	

1. In a bowl, combine anchovies, garlic, parsley, sauerkraut, capers, tarragon, mayonnaise and mustard. Season to taste with salt and pepper.

2. Use immediately or cover tightly and store in the refrigerator for up to 2 days.

Ketchup

*Yes, you can make your
own ketchup, and it tastes
even better than what
you get in a bottle! This
recipe uses honey as the
sweetener, which makes it
perfect for a Gapster.*

Tips

The amount of ketchup you
end up with depends on how
much you reduce it in step 4.

Unless you happen to have
a whole lot of small plastic
containers, you can freeze
ketchup in a couple of large
containers. Once frozen,
let the blocks thaw for
30 minutes, then cut them
into chunks of the desired
size. Refreeze in a large
freezer bag, making sure the
chunks don't touch or they
will stick together. Now you
can easily take out a small
amount at a time.

• *Blender*

2	stalks celery, chopped	2
1	clove garlic, minced	1
½	small onion, chopped	½
3 cups	crushed tomatoes (from a jar)	750 mL
1 tsp	salt (approx.)	5 mL
1 tbsp	honey	15 mL

Essence

3	whole cloves	3
1	bay leaf	1
1	1½-inch (4 cm) cinnamon stick	1
½ tsp	whole black peppercorns	2 mL
½ tsp	whole or ground allspice	2 mL
Pinch	cayenne pepper (optional)	Pinch
6 tbsp	white wine vinegar (approx.)	90 mL

1. In a medium pot, combine celery, garlic, onion, tomatoes and salt; bring to a simmer over medium-low heat. Reduce heat and simmer, stirring occasionally, for 30 minutes or until vegetables are soft.

2. *Essence:* Meanwhile, in a small saucepan, combine cloves, bay leaf, cinnamon stick, peppercorns, allspice, cayenne (if using) and vinegar; bring to a simmer over medium-low heat. Simmer for 15 minutes or until flavors are infused.

3. Transfer tomato mixture to blender and blend until smooth. Return to pot.

4. Strain essence through a sieve into tomato mixture; discard spices. Simmer over low heat, uncovered, stirring occasionally, until thickened as desired. (It may take a couple of hours. Keep an eye on it!)

5. Stir in honey, then taste and adjust seasoning as desired with salt and/or vinegar. Let cool.

Pesto

Pesto is delicious as a dip or with vegetables, fish or meat. When you are transitioning out of the GAPS diet, you may add it to a potato salad.

Tips

Use only the basil leaves and reserve the stems for juicing.

Store pesto in an airtight container in the refrigerator for up to 5 days or in the freezer for up to 6 months.

- **Blender**

2½ oz	dried soaked pine nuts (see page 74)	75 g
3	large handfuls basil leaves	3
1	large clove garlic, crushed	1
½ to ⅔ cup	cold-pressed olive oil	125 to 150 mL
¾ cup	freshly grated Parmesan cheese	175 mL
	Salt	

1. In blender, combine pine nuts, basil, garlic and ½ cup (150 mL) oil; blend until fairly smooth, adding more oil as necessary for the desired consistency.

2. Transfer to a bowl and stir in cheese. Season with salt (but cautiously, as Parmesan itself is salty).

Oil and Vinegar Dressing

*This classic dressing works
with all kinds of leafy greens
and other vegetables. Try
it on avocado with lightly
toasted pine nuts. Its flavor
improves as it sits in the
refrigerator.*

Tips

To vary the flavor, add
a drop of cold-pressed
pumpkin seed oil or another
tasty cold-pressed plant oil.

Store in the refrigerator for up
to 5 days. For longer storage,
omit the garlic, store the
dressing for up to 1 month
and add garlic up to 5 days
before serving.

1 cup	cold-pressed olive oil	250 mL
1 tbsp	no-added-sugar balsamic vinegar	15 mL
1½ tsp	Dijon mustard	7 mL
3	cloves garlic, halved	3
	Chopped fresh basil or dried thyme	

1. In a bowl, whisk together oil, vinegar and mustard until mustard is completely dissolved.

2. Pour dressing into a clean container with a lid. Add garlic and basil.

Jellied Broth

**Makes 1 cup
(250 mL)**

Jellied broth tastes amazing and helps maintain the body's cells. Eat it on your pâtés or with other cold meat dishes.

Tips

Choose a good-quality brand of unflavored gelatin powder made from grass-fed animals, such as Great Lakes or Vital Protein. Make sure to get the type of gelatin that can congeal, not the type meant only as a supplement. For more information, see page 55.

Jellied broth can be stored in an airtight container in the refrigerator for up to 5 days.

1 cup	Bone Broth (page 99)	250 mL
	Salt	
1½ tsp	unflavored gelatin powder	7 mL

1. In a small saucepan, heat broth over medium-high heat until steaming. Season to taste with salt.

2. Transfer broth to a bowl and sprinkle with gelatin, stirring to dissolve. Chill until set.

Snacks

Soft-Curd Cheese with Herbs

Makes 4 servings

This adaptation of soft-curd cheese is delicious with fresh radishes and as a dip for cucumbers and carrots. You can also use it as a sauce with meatballs, or as a sandwich spread once you are ready to transition out of the GAPS diet.

2 tbsp	chopped fresh parsley	30 mL
2 tbsp	snipped fresh chives	30 mL
2 tbsp	chopped fresh cilantro	30 mL
5 oz	Soft-Curd Cheese (page 71)	150 g
1½ tsp	cold-pressed olive oil	7 mL
½ tsp	salt	2 mL
	Freshly ground black pepper	

1. Reserve some of each of the parsley, chives and cilantro for garnish.

2. In a bowl, stir together the remaining parsley, chives and cilantro, cheese, olive oil and salt. Season to taste with pepper.

3. Serve sprinkled with the reserved herbs.

More GAPS Snacks

Other great snacks for the GAPS diet include cherry tomatoes, olives, carrots, nuts, fresh fruit, a glass of kefir or a chunk of cheese.

Spicy Soft-Curd Cheese

Makes 4 servings

Yet another take on soft-curd cheese! This one is good for lunch, as a dip or as an accompaniment for meatballs.

1	clove garlic, minced	1
5 oz	Soft-Curd Cheese (page 71)	150 g
½ to 1 tsp	salt	2 to 5 mL
¾ tsp	paprika	3 mL
¾ tsp	ground cumin	3 mL
1½ tsp	cold-pressed olive oil	7 mL
	Freshly ground black pepper	

1. In a bowl, stir together garlic, cheese, ½ tsp (2 mL) salt, paprika, cumin and oil. Season to taste with pepper and more salt, if necessary.

Marinated Sun-Dried Tomatoes

Makes 8 servings

Eat these plain, serve them with cheese or add them to Fish Lasagna (page 152).

Tip

If you wish to store the tomatoes for longer than 5 days, omit the garlic or add it a day or two before you plan to use the tomatoes.

- **2-cup (500 mL) glass jar**

2½ oz	dry-packed sun-dried tomatoes	75 g
	Boiling water	
5	cloves garlic	5
3 or 4	sprigs fresh basil	3 or 4
⅔ cup	cold-pressed olive oil (approx.)	150 mL

1. Place tomatoes in a bowl, cover with boiling water and let soak for about 1 hour, until soft. Drain tomatoes and pat dry.

2. In jar, layer tomatoes, garlic and basil. Pour in enough olive oil to cover completely. Cover and let marinate in the refrigerator for at least 1 day or up to 5 days.

Beet Chips

**Makes 4 to
6 servings**

*These chips are so crispy
and flavorful, you won't be
able to get enough of them.
It does take some time to
make them, though. Serve
them as a snack or for
dinner with a roast.*

Tips

This recipe will be time-
consuming and tedious if
you don't have a convection
oven; I don't recommend
attempting it in a regular
oven.

For very thin beet slices,
use a mandoline.

If you are able to keep from
eating these chips instantly,
you can store them for a
couple of days in an airtight
container. If they lose their
crispness, place them in
a 230°F (115°C) oven for
15 minutes.

- **Preheat convection oven to 230°F (115°C)**
- **3 baking sheets, lined with parchment paper**

$\frac{1}{4}$ to $\frac{1}{2}$ cup	duck, goose or chicken lard, Clarified Butter (page 68) or coconut oil	60 to 125 mL
2 lbs	beets (about 5 large), peeled and very thinly sliced (see tip)	1 kg
$\frac{1}{2}$ tsp	salt	2 mL

1. In a small saucepan, melt cooking fat over low heat. Let cool.

2. Place beets in a large bowl. Pour fat over beets and stir, making sure all the beets are completely coated in fat.

3. Arrange beet slices in a single layer on prepared baking sheets. You can place them close to one another, as they shrink.

4. Place all the baking sheets in the oven and bake for about $1\frac{1}{2}$ hours or until crispy. Be sure to keep an eye on them near the end, as they crisp quickly then.

5. Transfer chips to a platter and sprinkle with salt.

Sesame Crisps

**Makes 8 servings
(about 40 pieces)**

*Serve these as an
alternative to chips, with
one or more dips, such as
Pesto (page 191), Tomato
Salsa (page 87), Aïoli
(page 188), Spicy Soft-
Curd Cheese (page 196),
Guacamole (page 139)
or White Bean Hummus
(page 139).*

Tips

Sesame flour is available
online and at some well-
stocked health food stores.

If the crisps, against all odds,
do not become entirely crisp,
you can toast them after
breaking them into pieces for
3 to 4 minutes in the middle
of the oven.

The crisps can be stored
in an airtight container at
room temperature for up to
10 days.

- *Preheat oven to 350°F (180°C), with rack set in second-lowest
  position*
- *High-speed blender or food processor*
- *2 baking sheets, lined with parchment paper*

2	large eggs	2
6 tbsp	butter	90 mL
1⅓ cups	sesame flour	325 mL
½ tsp	salt	2 mL
2 tbsp	nigella seeds	30 mL

1. In blender, process eggs and butter until blended.
   Add flour and salt; process until a dense, spreadable
   dough forms.

2. Divide dough in half, then divide each half into fifths.
   Spread one portion as thinly as possible in a rectangle
   about 12 by 2½ inches (30 by 6 cm) on one of the baking
   sheets. (It is more important to spread the dough thinly
   than to measure precisely.) Make 5 rectangles on each
   baking sheet. Sprinkle nigella seeds on top.

3. Bake, one sheet at a time, in preheated oven for about
   12 minutes or until golden. Let cool on a wire rack.

4. Break rectangles into pieces the size of crackers or
   potato chips.

Almond and Seed Crackers

**Makes about
18 crackers**

*These crackers make a
great snack at any time
of day. Top them with
a GAPS-friendly cheese
or spread butter and a
bit of honey on top for
a cookie-like treat.*

Tips

The crackers will look best if
you have a cookie or biscuit
cutter to use as a mold; they
can be molded without a
cutter, but it can get pretty
messy and the crackers may
look rather strange; the flavor,
however, will be just as good.

The crisps can be stored
in an airtight container at
room temperature for up to
10 days.

- *2½-inch (6 cm) round cookie or biscuit cutter (see tip)*
- *Baking sheet, lined with parchment paper*

1⅔ oz	dried soaked almonds (see page 74), finely chopped	50 g
1⅔ oz	dried soaked pumpkin seeds, finely chopped	50 g
1⅔ oz	sesame seeds	50 g
1⅔ oz	flax seeds	50 g
½ tsp	salt	2 mL
1 tbsp	butter or Clarified Butter (page 68), melted	15 mL
1	large egg, beaten	1

1. In a bowl, combine almonds, pumpkin seeds, sesame seeds, flax seeds, salt and butter. Add egg and knead until incorporated. Let stand for 10 minutes.

3. Meanwhile, preheat oven to 350°F (180°C), with rack set in second-lowest position.

4. Place cookie cutter on prepared baking sheet. Spoon a heaping tablespoonful (15 mL) of dough into the ring. Pound with the handle of a wooden spoon to make an even layer inside the ring. Carefully loosen the ring and lift off to leave the circle of dough. Repeat, spacing crackers apart, until dough is used up.

5. Bake for 12 minutes or until light golden.

Salted Almonds

Makes 4 to 8 servings

A handful of salted nuts is a wonderful snack that is perfectly complemented by a glass of sparkling water or cold, dry cider. You can also add them to a buffet table or bring them with you on a picnic or a hike. They stay crisp for several days.

- *Preheat oven to 350°F (180°C), with rack set in second-lowest position*
- *Small ovenproof bowl*

3½ oz	dried soaked almonds (see page 74)	100 g
2 tbsp	Clarified Butter (page 68)	30 mL
¼ tsp	salt	1 mL

1. In ovenproof bowl, combine almonds and butter, stirring to coat evenly.

2. Bake in preheated oven, stirring occasionally, for about 20 minutes or until fragrant and browned.

3. Using a spoon, transfer almonds to a paper towel and sprinkle with salt. Serve warm or let cool.

Variation

You can replace the almonds with any kind of nut, such as hazelnuts, cashews or pistachios, as long as they have been soaked and dried as directed on page 74.

Beverages

Hot and Cold Drink Options

If you need something cold to drink other than filtered water, you can drink:

- Sparkling water with or without a touch of apple cider vinegar (from intro diet, stage 1)
- Vallentino's Favorite Drink (page 206) (from intro diet, stage 1)
- Freshly pressed vegetable juice (from intro diet, stage 4)
- Freshly pressed vegetable juice with some fruit juice (from intro diet, stage 5)
- Sparkling water with pure, unsweetened apple juice, in equal parts (from intro diet, stage 5)
- Sparkling water with a lemon slice (from intro diet, stage 6)
- Pure, unsweetened apple, pear or other fruit juice in moderate amounts (from intro diet, stage 6)

All with or without ice cubes!

In addition, look online (or in books) for recipes for fermented beverages like water kefir, kombucha and kvass.

Making Your Own Juices

Freshly pressed vegetable juices are not just refreshing and tasty, they are also a great source of vitamins, minerals and other micronutrients. In addition, they kickstart the detoxification process without any fiber to irritate the intestine. GAPS practitioners recommend juicing systematically from stage 4 of the intro diet, while on the full diet and afterward!

Store-bought juices will not help you detoxify, as they have been sterilized with either heat or high-pressure pasteurization, both of which kill microorganisms so efficiently that the beneficial nutrients are also destroyed.

Only your taste and imagination limit the possible combinations for making juice. I would like to emphasize, though: if you are using red beets, they should make up only 5% of the total amount, to avoid upsetting your digestive system. And if you're adding fruit juice for flavor and sweetness, use a maximum of 50% fruit juice.

Herbal Teas

It's not always clear what's actually in an herbal tea bag — it might contain ingredients that we don't want to consume on the GAPS diet. So look for pure, GAPS-friendly herbal teas or make your own!

Tip

All teas can be sweetened with a little honey, unless you are trying to control candida.

Ginger Tea

1 cup	boiling water	250 mL
4	thin slices gingerroot	4

1. In a tea cup, pour boiling water over ginger and let cool for a couple of minutes. Leave the slices in the cup.

Chamomile Tea

1 cup	boiling water	250 mL
1 tsp	dried chamomile flowers	5 mL

1. In a measuring cup or bowl, pour boiling water over chamomile flowers. Let steep for 6 minutes. Strain through a tea strainer or fine-mesh sieve into a tea cup.

Lemon Tea (Intro Diet, Stage 6)

1 cup	boiling water	250 mL
1	slice organic lemon	1

1. In a tea cup, pour boiling water over lemon. Leave the peel in the cup, or remove half for a less bitter flavor.

Teas for Boiling

- *Ipe Roxo Tea:* (Also known as Pau d'Arco tea or Lapacho tea.) Boil 1½ tbsp (22 mL) dried bark in 2 cups (500 mL) water for 15 minutes. Strain and drink. Store extra tea in the refrigerator and reheat to serve.

- *Turmeric Tea:* Boil 1 tsp (5 mL) ground turmeric in 3⅔ cups (900 mL) water for 10 minutes. Drain through a coffee filter and drink. Store extra tea in the refrigerator and reheat to serve.

Vallentino's Favorite Drink

Makes 1 serving

This refreshing, sparkling probiotic drink is pure luxury on a hot summer day.

Tips

Regulate the amount of whey according to your own process. If you are just beginning the diet, avoid severe die-off symptoms (see page 26) by starting with a very small amount of probiotics (consult with your GAPS practitioner about the dosage), then gradually increasing it.

Yogurt whey, which is slightly less potent than kefir whey, can be substituted.

1 cup	sparkling water	250 mL
1 tsp	apple cider vinegar	5 mL
½ tsp to 2 tbsp	kefir whey (see page 94)	2 to 30 mL

1. In a glass, combine sparkling water, vinegar and whey (see tip); stir together and serve immediately.

Carrot Juice

Makes 1 serving

Carrot juice tastes wonderful when freshly pressed, it is mild on your digestion, and it has an excellent therapeutic effect.

Tip

If you peel the carrots, you can reserve the pulp and use it for baking.

- **Juicer**

1 lb	carrots	500 g
	Fresh parsley stems (optional)	
	Finely grated gingerroot	

1. Juice carrots and parsley stems (if using) according to manufacturer's directions.

2. Place ginger to taste in a glass and pour in juice; stir and serve immediately.

Carrot Coconut Juice

Makes 1 serving

Freshly made vegetable juice is such a treat. It's filling, it's refreshing, and it's full of good stuff.

Tip

You can also make coconut water by soaking 2 tbsp (30 mL) unsweetened coarsely shredded coconut overnight in ½ cup (125 mL) water and straining it. Reserve the water! You need about ½ cup (125 mL) coconut water for this recipe. If you are on the full diet, you can dry the strained coconut and use it for baking.

- **Juicer**

1	coconut (see tip)	1
10 oz	carrots	300 g
¼ tsp	grated gingerroot	1 mL

1. Break open the coconut and pour the coconut water into a container. (If you are on the full diet, you can shred the coconut meat and use it to make Coconut Milk, page 76, or dry it for use in baked goods.)

2. Juice carrots according to manufacturer's directions. Stir coconut water into carrot juice.

3. Place ginger in a glass and pour in juice; stir and serve immediately.

Green Juice

Makes 1 serving

Green juices can help relieve certain GAPS-related conditions. You can customize the juice to your taste by using any type of green vegetables you prefer.

- **Juicer**

5	leaves baby romaine lettuce (including stems)	5
1	large handful spinach (about ⅔ oz/20 g)	1
1	4- to 6-inch (10 to 15 cm) cucumber	1
½ tsp	grated gingerroot	2 mL

1. Juice romaine, spinach and cucumber according to manufacturer's directions.

2. Place ginger in a glass and pour in juice; stir and serve immediately.

Carrot, Apple and Celery Juice

Makes 1 serving

You don't need all sorts of fancy ingredients to make a really tasty freshly pressed juice. Enjoy this delightful concoction as it is or, for a more filling drink, add it to a smoothie (see page 209).

- **Juicer**

7 oz	carrots	200 g
7 oz	apples	200 g
1	stalk celery	1
1/4 tsp	grated gingerroot	1 mL

1. Juice carrots, apples and celery according to manufacturer's directions.

2. Place ginger in a glass and pour in juice; stir and serve immediately.

Variation

You can use other vegetables, such as celery root, parsley stalks, cucumbers, lettuce or spinach. If you use red beets, they should make up a maximum of 5% of the total weight, to avoid upsetting your digestive system.

GAPS Smoothie

Makes 1 serving

The fat in eggs, sour cream, butter and coconut oil has a stabilizing effect on blood sugar, reducing the effect of fresh juices on your blood sugar levels.

Tips

Publisher's note: Although raw eggs are considered nourishing in the GAPS diet, they may contain salmonella (see sidebar, page 22). If you prefer to err on the side of caution, you can replace the egg in this recipe with 3 tbsp (45 mL) pasteurized liquid whole egg or simply use a pasteurized in-shell egg, if available. Note that, while pasteurized eggs are not part of the GAPS nutritional protocol, food safety must be your first priority.

If you cannot tolerate egg whites, use 2 large egg yolks in place of the whole egg.

¾ cup	freshly pressed vegetable juice (pages 206–208)	175 mL
1	large egg (see tips)	1
1 to 2 tbsp	Sour Cream (page 92), butter or coconut oil	15 to 30 mL
	Grated gingerroot (optional)	

1. In a glass, whisk together vegetable juice, egg and the desired amount of sour cream. Stir in ginger to taste (if using) and serve immediately.

Carrot and Avocado Smoothie

Makes 1 serving

This is a very GAPS-friendly drink — detoxifying, pro-biotic, tasty and satisfying!

Variation
You can use other vegetables, such as celery, celery root, cucumbers or spinach. If you use red beets, they should make up a maximum of 5% of the total weight, to avoid upsetting your digestive system.

- **Juicer**
- **Blender**

3²/₃ oz	carrots	110 g
½	apple (about 1²/₃ oz/50 g)	½
¼ cup	Kefir (page 94)	60 mL
½	ripe avocado	½
½	ripe banana	½
	Grated gingerroot	

1. Juice carrots and apple according to manufacturer's directions.

2. In blender, combine juice, kefir, avocado and banana; purée until smooth.

3. Pour into a glass and stir in ginger to taste. Serve immediately.

Strawberry Smoothie

Makes 1 serving

Frozen strawberries give this smoothie a thick texture and make it delightfully cold. But you can use fresh strawberries instead, if you have them on hand.

Tips
In recipes that are not heated, use raw honey for its added health benefits.

If using vanilla extract, check the label to make sure it contains only vanilla, water and alcohol, with no other additives.

- **Blender**

3½ oz	frozen strawberries, halved	100 g
1	ripe banana	1
²/₃ cup	Kefir (page 94)	150 mL
½ tsp	raw honey	2 mL
½ tsp	Vanilla Vodka (page 79) or pure vanilla extract	2 mL
¼ tsp	grated lime or lemon zest	1 mL

1. In blender, combine strawberries, banana, kefir, honey, vanilla vodka and lime zest; purée until smooth.

2. Pour into a glass and serve immediately.

Kefir Eggnog

Makes 1 serving

Eggnog is typically made with buttermilk, but kefir, which tastes like buttermilk, which is GAPS-friendly and has probiotic benefits, can easily be used in its place.

Tips

Publisher's note: Although raw eggs are considered nourishing in the GAPS diet, they may contain salmonella (see sidebar, page 22). If you prefer to err on the side of caution, you can replace the egg yolk in this recipe with 1½ tbsp (22 mL) pasteurized liquid whole egg or simply use the yolk from a pasteurized in-shell egg, if available. Note that, while pasteurized eggs are not part of the GAPS nutritional protocol, food safety must be your first priority.

Bake Archipelago Macaroons (page 254) and serve them as an accompaniment.

1	large egg yolk (see tip)	1
1½ tsp	raw honey	7 mL
Pinch	vanilla seeds from a split bean	Pinch
	Grated lemon zest	
1 cup	Kefir (page 94)	250 mL

1. In a bowl, whisk egg yolk and honey vigorously until pale and thickened. (It takes longer than when using sugar.) Whisk in vanilla seeds, a touch of lemon zest and kefir until blended.

2. Pour into a tall glass and serve immediately.

Mulled Wine

Makes 4 to
5 servings

Hot, spicy wine is a nice treat when it's cold outside. In this recipe, the wine is flavored with just a few spices, citrus fruits and honey, so it's fairly easy to make.

Tip

Keep the cooked orange pieces in the mulled wine when you're pouring it into glasses; they taste nice.

• *Colander lined with a lint-free tea towel or several layers of cheesecloth*

1 cup	water	250 mL
2½ tbsp	honey	37 mL
12	whole cloves	12
1	2-inch (5 cm) cinnamon stick	1
	Zest of ½ lemon (peeled with a vegetable peeler)	
¼ tsp	finely grated nutmeg	1 mL
1	orange (unpeeled), cut into 24 chunks	1
1	bottle (750 mL) dry red wine	1

1. In a medium saucepan, combine water, honey, cloves, cinnamon, lemon zest and nutmeg; cover and bring to a boil over medium-high heat. Reduce heat to low and simmer for 10 minutes.

2. Pour liquid through lined colander into a measuring cup or bowl, discarding solids.

3. Return liquid to saucepan and add half the orange pieces; bring to a boil over medium-high heat. Reduce heat and simmer for 1 minute.

4. Add red wine and heat over medium heat until liquid reaches 175°F to 200°F (80°C to 90°C). Do not let boil. Remove from heat.

5. Divide the remaining orange pieces among cups or heat-resistant glasses; pour in mulled wine. If desired, place a long teaspoon in each glass. Serve immediately.

Mulled Apple Cider

Makes 5 servings

Apple cider is very sweet, so there is hardly any honey or other sweetener in this recipe. If you are lucky enough to have access to an apple tree with juicy apples — and you tolerate fruit sugar — you can juice them to make the cider.

Tip

Keep the cooked orange pieces in the mulled cider when you're pouring it into glasses; they taste nice.

- *Colander lined with a lint-free tea towel or several layers of cheesecloth*

1 cup	water	250 mL
1 tsp	honey	5 mL
5	whole cloves	5
1	1-inch (2.5 cm) cinnamon stick	1
	Zest of ½ lemon (peeled with a vegetable peeler)	
¼ tsp	finely grated nutmeg	1 mL
1	orange (unpeeled), cut into 24 chunks	1
4 cups	unsweetened apple cider	1 L

1. In a medium saucepan, combine water, honey, cloves, cinnamon, lemon zest and nutmeg; cover and bring to a boil over medium-high heat. Reduce heat to low and simmer for 10 minutes.

2. Pour liquid through lined colander into a measuring cup or bowl, discarding solids.

3. Return liquid to saucepan and add 14 of the orange pieces; bring to a boil over medium-high heat. Reduce heat and simmer for 1 minute.

4. Add apple cider and heat over medium heat until liquid reaches 175°F to 200°F (80°C to 90°C). Do not let boil. Remove from heat.

5. Divide the remaining orange pieces among cups or heat-resistant glasses; pour in mulled cider and serve immediately.

Sweets

Banana Pancakes

Makes 2 pancakes

2	large eggs	2
1	ripe banana, mashed	1
	Butter, Clarified Butter (page 68) or coconut oil	

These pancakes are great for breakfast or dessert. Serve them with fresh fruit, Applesauce (page 219), berry coulis, Orange Sauce (page 266), ice cream (page 231), Coconut Whipped Cream (page 261), Sour Cream (page 92) or anything you like!

1. In a bowl, whisk eggs and banana until blended.

2. In a medium skillet or crêpe pan, melt a generous layer of cooking fat over medium heat. Pour in half the egg mixture and cook for 3 to 5 minutes or until golden on the bottom. Remove pancake from skillet (see tip), add more fat to skillet, then invert pancake back into skillet. Cook for about 3 minutes or until pancake is set and golden.

3. Repeat step 2 with the remaining egg mixture, adding more fat and adjusting heat as necessary between pancakes.

Tips

A crêpe pan's low edges make it easier to flip flourless pancakes, and a crêpe spatula (an oblong palette knife, usually made of wood) will make it easier to flip them.

To easily remove the pancake from the skillet and turn it over, use a crêpe spatula to slide the pancake onto a lid, then invert it back into the skillet.

These pancakes taste great drizzled with a little melted butter or coconut oil mixed with raw honey and ground cinnamon.

Sour Cream Pancakes

Makes 2 pancakes

Eggs, full-fat sour cream and butter or coconut oil — that's GAPS-friendly food! These pancakes aren't just a delicious dessert; they keep my daughter going from morning until lunch every day, and she enjoys every mouthful.

Tips

If you have raw honey, don't add it to the batter; drizzle it over the cooked pancakes instead, so its nutrients aren't destroyed by the cooking process.

Serve with fresh fruit, Applesauce (page 219), berry coulis, Orange Sauce (page 266), ice cream (page 231), Coconut Whipped Cream (page 261) or Sour Cream (page 92).

2	large eggs	2
1 tbsp	Sour Cream (page 92)	15 mL
	A drop of honey (optional)	
	Butter, Clarified Butter (page 68) or coconut oil	

1. In a bowl, whisk eggs, sour cream and honey (if using) until blended.

2. In a medium skillet or crêpe pan, melt a generous layer of cooking fat over medium heat. Pour in half the egg mixture and cook for 1 to 2 minutes or until golden brown on the bottom. Remove pancake from skillet (see tip, page 216), add more fat to skillet, then invert pancake back into skillet. Cook for 1 to 2 minutes or until pancake is set and golden brown. (If they contain honey, the pancakes will brown more quickly, so keep an eye on them!)

3. Repeat step 2 with the remaining egg mixture, adding more fat and adjusting heat as necessary between pancakes.

Variation

For a luxury edition when you are on the full GAPS diet, add a couple of drops of Vanilla Vodka (page 79) or pure vanilla extract to the batter.

Honey Apple Waffles

Makes 8 waffles

I started experimenting with making GAPS-friendly waffles when I got hold of an unused secondhand electric waffle maker for less than 6 dollars. A few batches later, I was delighted with the results. These naturally sweet waffles are especially nice on a cold day, and make a great breakfast-on-the-go too.

Tips

The waffle maker should be quite hot before the batter is poured in.

If using vanilla extract, check the label to make sure it contains only vanilla, water and alcohol, with no other additives.

- **Nut grinder (see box, page 75)**
- **Electric mixer**
- **Electric waffle maker**

2½ oz	dried soaked almonds (see page 74)	75 g
7 oz	grated peeled apples	200 g
Pinch	salt	Pinch
4	large egg yolks	4
¼ cup	honey	60 mL
1 to 2 tsp	Vanilla Vodka (page 79) or pure vanilla extract	5 to 10 mL
6	large egg whites	6
1 tsp	honey	5 mL
¼ cup	melted coconut oil	60 mL
	Additional coconut oil	

1. In nut grinder, grind almonds into fine flour.

2. In a large bowl, combine almond flour, apples and salt, stirring well.

3. In a medium bowl, whisk egg yolks and ¼ cup (60 mL) honey vigorously until pale and thickened. (It takes longer than if you were using sugar.) Stir in vanilla vodka to taste.

4. In another medium bowl, using electric mixer, beat egg whites until very stiff, drizzling in 1 tsp (5 mL) honey halfway through for stabilization.

5. Preheat waffle maker (see tip).

6. Add egg yolk mixture to almond flour mixture, stirring until well combined. Stir in melted coconut oil. Carefully fold in one-quarter of the egg whites, then another quarter, then the remaining half.

7. Brush hot waffle maker with coconut oil. Ladle in batter and cook according to manufacturer's directions until golden. Repeat with remaining batter, brushing waffle maker with coconut oil as necessary between waffles.

Applesauce

**Makes about
6 cups (1.5 L)**

*Wonderful with coconut
cake, in a trifle, with
pancakes, with sour cream
or just as it is.*

Tips

Choose an apple variety that
doesn't require sweetening
but isn't too sour, such
as Fuji, Golden Delicious,
Gravenstein, Jonagold or
McIntosh.

To store the applesauce,
transfer it to an airtight
container and return the
vanilla bean to the sauce.
Store in the refrigerator for
up to 1 week. When the
applesauce is used up, let
the vanilla bean dry. It can
be used again.

You can also freeze the
applesauce in smaller
portions for up to 1 year.

- *Juicer*

4 lbs	apples	2 kg
	Cold water	
½ to 1	vanilla bean, split	½ to 1

1. Quarter apples and reserve cores.

2. In juicer, process apple cores. Measure the amount of juice and add enough cold water to make 7 tbsp (105 mL) liquid.

3. In a saucepan, combine apples, vanilla bean and apple juice; bring to a simmer over medium-high heat. Reduce heat to low, cover and simmer, stirring occasionally, for about 30 minutes or until mixture is the consistency of a purée. Let cool.

4. Remove vanilla bean (see tip) and strain purée through a sieve, discarding skins.

Variation

Substitute 1 tbsp (15 mL) Vanilla Vodka (page 79) or pure vanilla extract for the vanilla bean.

Rhubarb Compote

Makes about
3¼ cups (800 mL)

This tasty fruit treat is good simply topped with yogurt, sour cream or ice cream, or spooned over pancakes or waffles.

Tips

Use a large chef's knife to cut the rhubarb.

Leave the vanilla bean in the compote until you're serving it, then remove it and dry it for later reuse.

- **4- to 6-cup (1 to 1.5 L) shallow baking dish**

⅔ cup	honey	150 mL
½	vanilla bean, split and scraped	½
	Grated zest and juice of ¼ lemon	
1 lb	rhubarb stalks (without leaves)	500 g

1. In ovenproof dish, combine honey, vanilla bean and seeds, lemon zest and lemon juice.
2. Rinse rhubarb and remove brown areas. Pat stalks dry and cut into ¾-inch (2 cm) pieces.
3. Add rhubarb to honey mixture, stirring to coat, and marinate at room temperature for at least 2 hours or overnight.
4. Preheat oven to 400°F (200°C), with rack set in second-lowest position.
5. Bake rhubarb for 20 minutes, stirring occasionally, until rhubarb is tender but still retains its shape. Let cool.

Variation

Substitute 2 tsp (10 mL) Vanilla Vodka (page 79) or pure vanilla extract for the vanilla bean.

Plum Compote

Makes 4 to
6 servings

This compote goes best with homemade sour cream to balance the sweet flavor of the plums and honey. But if you cannot tolerate sour cream, enjoy it with coconut whipped cream instead.

Tip

If using vanilla extract, check the label to make sure it contains only vanilla, water and alcohol, with no other additives.

6	ripe plums (about 12 oz/375 g total), quartered	6
8 tsp	honey	40 mL
2 tsp	Vanilla Vodka (page 79) or pure vanilla extract	10 mL
1 tsp	freshly squeezed lemon juice	5 mL
4 to 6 tbsp	Sour Cream (page 92) or Coconut Whipped Cream (page 261)	60 to 90 mL
1	recipe Hazelnut Croquant (page 267), made with cinnamon	1

1. Place plums in a pot and add honey, vanilla vodka and lemon juice. Let marinate for about 1 hour to dissolve the honey.

2. Bring plum mixture to a simmer over low heat. Simmer for 2 to 5 minutes, depending on how tender you want them.

3. Divide plum compote equally among four to six dessert bowls. Top each with 1 tbsp (15 mL) sour cream and garnish with croquant.

Honeyed Pears

Makes 4 servings

Serve this attractive dish as is with a piece of blue cheese, or with Sour Cream (page 92), Coconut Whipped Cream (page 261), Kefir Eggnog (page 211) or Honey Nut Ice Cream (page 231).

Tips

The poaching liquid can also be used as a syrup for cakes, such as Coconut Cake (page 244).

To store the cooled pears, sterilize a 3-cup (750 mL) mason jar in scalding water, then rinse well with 1 tbsp (15 mL) Vanilla Vodka (page 79). Carefully transfer pears to jar and cover with marinade. Cover jar with lid and store in the refrigerator for up to 3 weeks. Garnish with nuts just before serving.

• *3-cup (750 mL) mason jar (optional)*

1²/₃ cups	water	400 mL
¹/₂ cup	honey	125 mL
	Grated zest of 1 lemon	
	Juice of ¹/₄ to ¹/₂ lemon	
¹/₂	vanilla bean, split	¹/₂
4	pears, peeled and halved lengthwise	4
	Handful chopped walnuts or toasted almonds (see page 74)	

1. In a large, wide saucepan, combine water, honey, lemon zest, lemon juice to taste and vanilla bean; bring to a boil over medium heat.

2. Carefully spoon halved pears into marinade and return to a boil. Reduce heat and simmer for 2 minutes or until slightly softened but not too soft.

3. Let pears cool completely in marinade. Serve garnished with walnuts.

Baked Apples

This dessert has been popular for time immemorial in regions all around the world. It's a cozy favorite on a cold day but is also delightful at a campfire (see variation). Serve warm with Sour Cream (page 92) or Coconut Whipped Cream (page 261).

Tips

Use large apples that are easy to hollow, such as Braeburn, Cortland, Empire, Granny Smith or Honeycrisp.

Reserve the apple lids for your next batch of juice.

You may vary the filling endlessly as long as you use GAPS-friendly ingredients.

- *Preheat oven to 350°F (180°C), with rack set in second-lowest position*
- *Baking dish, greased with butter or coconut oil*

2	large apples	2

Raisin Filling

1/3 oz	dried soaked almonds (see page 74), coarsely chopped	10 g
	Small handful raisins	
2 tsp	unsweetened coarsely shredded coconut	10 mL
1 tsp	ground cinnamon	5 mL
5 tsp	butter	25 mL
3 to 4 tsp	honey	15 to 20 mL

1. Using a paring knife, cut off an inverted cone–shaped lid from each apple (see tip). Hollow out the inside and remove the core, without cutting all the way through to the bottom. Place upright in prepared baking dish. (You may want to level the bottoms, so that the apples stand upright without tilting.)

2. *Raisin Filling:* In a small bowl, using a fork, stir together almonds, raisins, coconut, cinnamon, butter and honey to taste. Pack filling into apples.

3. Bake in preheated oven for 20 to 25 minutes or until apples are tender but still hold their shape. Let cool for 10 minutes and serve warm.

Variations

Hazelnut Filling: Replace the almonds with 1/2 oz (15 g) dried soaked hazelnuts, chopped, omit the raisins and replace the butter with coconut oil.

Cook the apples in a campfire instead of the oven. Wrap each filled apple in a double layer of foil and place them in the embers. Keep an eye on them; they may need less baking time than in the oven.

Ebelskivers

**Makes 20 to
24 ebelskivers**

*Serve ebelskivers alone
or with Orange Sauce
(page 266), a drop of
Vanilla Honey (page 78),
Strawberries in Honey
(page 265) or fresh berries.*

Tip

If using vanilla extract, check
the label to make sure it
contains only vanilla, water
and alcohol, with no other
additives.

- **Nut grinder (see box, page 75)**
- **Electric mixer**
- **7-well ebelskiver pan**

3½ oz	dried soaked hazelnuts (see page 74)	100 g
3	large eggs, separated	3
2 tbsp	honey	30 mL
½ tsp	ground cinnamon	2 mL
Pinch	salt	Pinch
1 tsp	Vanilla Vodka (page 79) or pure vanilla extract	5 mL
1	large cooking apple, peeled and finely diced	1
1 tsp	honey	5 mL
	Coconut oil or Clarified Butter (page 68)	

1. In nut grinder, grind hazelnuts into fine flour.

2. In a large bowl, whisk egg yolks and 2 tbsp (30 mL) honey vigorously until pale and thickened. Whisk in cinnamon, salt and vanilla vodka. Fold in apple and nut flour.

3. In another bowl, using electric mixer, beat egg whites until very stiff, drizzling in 1 tsp (5 mL) honey halfway through for stabilization.

4. Using a silicone spatula, carefully fold one-quarter of the egg white mixture into apple mixture. Fold in another quarter, then the remaining half.

5. Heat ebelskiver pan over medium-low heat and place 1 tsp (5 mL) cooking fat in each well. Pour about 2 tbsp (30 mL) batter into each well and cook for 3 to 4 minutes or until bottoms are light golden brown. Turn ebelskivers with a fork and cook for 3 to 4 minutes or until light golden brown on all sides. Transfer to a plate. Repeat with remaining batter, adding more fat and adjusting heat as necessary between batches.

Apple Jelly with Berries and Coconut Whipped Cream

Makes 4 servings

Fruit jelly is very healing, as long as you use gelatin made from grass-fed animals. Coconut whipped cream also provides good stuff for body and mind.

Tips

You can, of course, also make dessert jellies from other pure, unsweetened fruit juices.

Choose a good-quality brand of unflavored gelatin powder made from grass-fed animals, such as Great Lakes or Vital Protein. Make sure to get the type of gelatin that can congeal, not the type meant only as a supplement. For more information, see page 55.

- *Candy or instant-read thermometer*
- *4 clear glass dessert bowls*

2½ cups	unsweetened apple cider, divided	625 mL
8 tsp	unflavored gelatin powder	40 mL
28	raspberries or other sweet berries	28
	Coconut Whipped Cream (page 261)	

1. In a small pot, heat 1⅔ cups (400 mL) cider over low heat to 158°F to 176°F (70°C to 80°C).

2. Sprinkle gelatin in the remaining cider, whisking vigorously. Let stand for 1 minute, then whisk into warm cider, heating until gelatin is completely dissolved and liquid is clear.

3. Place a berry at the bottom of each of four dessert bowls. Cover with one-third of the cider mixture and let set in the freezer for 10 minutes.

4. Add 2 berries to each bowl and pour in another third of the cider. Let set in the freezer for 10 minutes.

5. Add 3 berries to each bowl and pour the remaining apple cider on top. Refrigerate for at least 30 minutes before serving or cover and refrigerate for up to 1 day.

6. Garnish each portion with coconut whipped cream and 1 raspberry.

Fruit Salad Deluxe

*Serve fruit salad with Sour
Cream (page 92), cold
Coconut Whipped Cream
(page 261) or Honey Nut
Ice Cream (page 231). It's
a nice choice for a party
buffet and can easily be
halved or doubled.*

Tips

If using vanilla extract, check
the label to make sure it
contains only vanilla, water
and alcohol, with no other
additives.

When toasting chopped
nuts, keep in mind that small
pieces can get semiburnt
before the bigger pieces
turn golden. When the small
pieces are nicely toasted,
remove them by sifting them
through a coarse strainer,
then finish toasting the
remaining big pieces.

Syrup

	Juice of $1/2$ lime	
	Grated zest and juice of $1/2$ orange	
1	drop Vanilla Vodka (page 79) or pure vanilla extract	1
1 tbsp	honey (preferably acacia honey)	15 mL

Fruit Salad

2 to 3	handfuls dried soaked hazelnuts (see page 74), coarsely chopped	2 to 3
2	apples, diced	2
1	pear, diced	1
$1\frac{1}{2}$	oranges	$1\frac{1}{2}$
30	seedless grapes	30
2	kiwifruits	2
2	bananas	2
2	handfuls blueberries	2

1. *Syrup:* In a small saucepan, combine lime juice, orange zest, orange juice, vanilla vodka and honey; cook over medium-low heat until reduced by half. Let cool.

2. *Fruit Salad:* Heat a dry skillet over medium heat. Spread hazelnuts in a single layer in the pan and cook, stirring often to avoid burning, for 3 to 4 minutes or until golden brown. Immediately transfer nuts to a plate, spread out in a single layer and let cool.

3. In a large serving bowl, combine apples and pear. Pour in syrup and stir gently to coat; let soak while you prepare the remaining fruit.

4. Peel oranges, remove the white membranes and dice the flesh. Halve grapes and dice kiwis and bananas.

5. Add oranges, grapes, kiwis, bananas and blueberries to apples and pears, stirring gently to coat. Sprinkle fruit salad with toasted nuts.

Raspberry Mousse

Makes 6 servings

This dessert is a treat all year round. When they're in season, you can use fresh berries in place of frozen, and if you can't get your hands on freeze-dried raspberries for the garnish, you can top each dessert with a fresh or thawed frozen raspberry.

Tips

Publisher's note: Although raw eggs are considered nourishing in the GAPS diet, they may contain salmonella (see sidebar, page 22). If you prefer to err on the side of caution, use pasteurized in-shell eggs, if they are available in your area. Note that, while pasteurized eggs are not part of the GAPS nutritional protocol, food safety must be your first priority.

If you have any leftovers, you can freeze the mousse, though it will taste a bit more sour when eaten frozen or partially frozen. Serve it with a bit of Kefir Eggnog (page 211) or a sweet cookie, such as an Almond Tuile (page 252) or a Florentine (page 253) without buttercream. You should remove the mousse from the freezer 30 to 45 minutes before serving it.

- *Blender*
- *Electric mixer*

2	large eggs, separated (see tip)	2
8 tsp	honey	40 mL
4 oz	frozen raspberries	125 g
2 tsp	Vanilla Vodka (page 79) or pure vanilla extract	10 mL
1 tsp	freshly squeezed lemon juice	5 mL
2 tsp	unflavored gelatin powder	10 mL
	Freeze-dried raspberries (see tip)	

1. In a large bowl, whisk egg yolks and honey vigorously until pale and thickened. (It takes longer than if you were using sugar.)

2. In blender, purée frozen raspberries until smooth.

3. In another medium bowl, using electric mixer, beat egg whites until stiff.

4. In your smallest saucepan, heat vanilla vodka and lemon juice over low heat. Sprinkle in gelatin, whisking, and heat until dissolved.

5. Whisk vodka mixture into egg yolk mixture, then quickly stir in puréed berries until smooth. Quickly but carefully fold in egg whites.

6. Spoon mousse into six dessert bowls. Cover and refrigerate for at least 1 hour or up to 24 hours. Serve garnished with freeze-dried raspberries.

Cocoa Mousse

This is one of very few recipes containing raw, sugar-free cocoa powder. If you are lucky enough to tolerate it, go ahead and indulge!

Tips

In recipes that are not heated, use raw honey for its added health benefits.

In place of the vanilla vodka, you can use the seeds from ⅛ vanilla bean.

When toasting chopped nuts, keep in mind that small pieces can get semiburnt before the bigger pieces turn golden. When the small pieces are nicely toasted, remove them by sifting them through a coarse strainer, then finish toasting the remaining big pieces.

• *Blender*

	Small handful dried soaked almonds (see page 74), coarsely chopped	
2	ripe bananas	2
3 tbsp	Sour Cream (page 92)	45 mL
2 tbsp	unsweetened cocoa powder	30 mL
2 tbsp	raw honey	30 mL
2 tsp	almond butter	10 mL
1 to 2 tsp	Vanilla Vodka (page 79)	5 to 10 mL

1. Heat a dry skillet over medium heat. Spread almonds in a single layer in the pan and cook, stirring often to avoid burning, for 3 to 4 minutes or until golden brown. Immediately transfer nuts to a plate, spread out in a single layer and let cool.

2. In blender, combine bananas, sour cream, cocoa, honey, almond butter and vanilla vodka to taste; purée until smooth.

3. Spoon mousse into dessert bowls and sprinkle with toasted almonds. Serve immediately.

Apple Cream

Makes 6 servings

This dessert was inspired by a recipe from the 19th century, a time when the use of sugar was beginning to increase. In this GAPS-friendly version, of course, honey is the sweetener.

Tip

Choose a good-quality brand of unflavored gelatin powder made from grass-fed animals, such as Great Lakes or Vital Protein. For more information, see page 55.

1 lb	apples, quartered	500 g
1	vanilla bean, split	1
²⁄₃ cup	dry white wine	150 mL
4	large egg yolks	4
8 tsp	honey	40 mL
1 tsp	freshly squeezed lemon juice	5 mL
1½ tsp	unflavored gelatin powder	7 mL
2	handfuls dried soaked hazelnuts or almonds (see page 74), chopped and lightly toasted	2
6	dried crisp apple rings	6

1. In a large saucepan, combine quartered apples, vanilla bean and wine. Bring to a simmer over medium heat. Reduce heat to low, cover and simmer, stirring occasionally, for about 30 minutes or until mixture is the consistency of a purée.

2. Remove vanilla bean and strain purée through a sieve, discarding skins.

3. In a large bowl, whisk egg yolks and honey vigorously until pale and thickened. (It takes longer than if you were using sugar.) Stir in apple purée and lemon juice.

4. Return apple mixture to pot and bring to a boil over medium-low heat, whisking constantly. Remove from heat and sprinkle in gelatin, whisking until dissolved.

5. Spoon apple cream into six dessert bowls. Let cool for at least 1 hour and leave in a cool place for up to 2 hours or refrigerate for up to 24 hours.

6. Just before serving, sprinkle each dessert with hazelnuts and stand an apple ring upright on top.

Almond Cream

Makes 4 to 5 servings

This is a delicious way to get your probiotics! Once you're in stage 6 of the intro diet, you can serve it with strawberries, cherries or raspberries in honey (page 265).

Tips

Publisher's note: Although raw eggs are considered nourishing in the GAPS diet, they may contain salmonella (see sidebar, page 22). If you prefer to err on the side of caution, use a pasteurized in-shell egg, if they are available in your area. Note that, while pasteurized eggs are not part of the GAPS nutritional protocol, food safety must be your first priority.

When toasting chopped nuts, keep in mind that small pieces can get semiburnt before the bigger pieces turn golden. When the small pieces are nicely toasted, remove them by sifting them through a coarse strainer, then finish toasting the remaining big pieces.

Prepare Sour Cream a couple of days in advance so it has time to set. You can substitute Coconut Kefir (page 93), which should also be made in advance.

- *Electric mixer*

1²/₃ oz	dried soaked almonds (see page 74), blanched and coarsely chopped	50 g
1	large egg, separated (see tip)	1
1½ tbsp	raw honey	22 mL
	Seeds from ½ vanilla bean	
1 tsp	unflavored gelatin powder	5 mL
2 tbsp	Sour Cream (page 92)	30 mL

1. Heat a dry skillet over medium heat. Spread almonds in a single layer in the pan and cook, stirring often to avoid burning, for 3 to 4 minutes or until golden brown. Immediately transfer nuts to a plate, spread out in a single layer and let cool. Reserve some nuts for garnish.

2. In a large bowl, whisk egg yolk and honey vigorously until pale and thickened. (It takes longer than if you were using sugar.) Fold in almonds and vanilla seeds.

3. In a medium bowl, using electric mixer, beat egg white until stiff.

4. Sprinkle egg yolk mixture with gelatin, whisking. Fold in sour cream. Using a silicone spatula, fold in egg white.

5. Spoon almond cream into four or five dessert bowls. Freeze for at least 2 hours or up to 24 hours. Remove from freezer 5 to 10 minutes before serving and sprinkle with the reserved almonds.

Variation

Add ½ tsp (2 mL) finely grated lemon zest to the egg yolk mixture with the sour cream. This option is suitable from stage 6 of the intro diet.

Honey Nut Ice Cream

Makes 4 servings

There are very few GAPS-friendly ice creams on the market — a good reason to make your own deliciously nutty version!

Tips

Publisher's note: Although raw eggs are considered nourishing in the GAPS diet, they may contain salmonella (see sidebar, page 22). If you prefer to err on the side of caution, you can replace the raw egg whites in this recipe with ½ cup (125 mL) pasteurized liquid egg whites or simply use the whites from pasteurized in-shell eggs, if available. Note that, while pasteurized eggs are not part of the GAPS nutritional protocol, food safety must be your first priority.

Homemade ice cream turns out best in an ice cream maker, but since this recipe contains very stiffly beaten egg whites, it keeps its shape during freezing even without one.

The ice cream can be stored in the freezer for up to 3 months.

- *Electric mixer*
- *Ice cream maker (optional)*

4	large egg whites (see tip)	4
2 tbsp	raw honey	30 mL
3½ oz	dried soaked walnuts, hazelnuts or cashews (see page 74), chopped	100 g
2⅔ cups	Coconut Milk (page 76)	400 mL

1. In a large bowl, using electric mixer, beat egg whites until partially stiff. Drizzle in honey and beat for about 10 minutes or until very stiff. Fold in nuts. Using a silicone spatula, gently fold in coconut milk (it must not separate).

2. Transfer to ice cream maker and freeze according to manufacturer's instructions, or pour into an airtight container and freeze until firm, about 6 hours.

Quick Strawberry Ice Cream

Makes 2 servings

This easy ice cream is delicious all by itself or as an accompaniment to Banana Mazarin Cake (page 243) or Coconut Cake (page 244).

Tips

Use a frozen banana for firmer ice cream or a fresh one for softer ice cream.

If you can't find freeze-dried strawberries for the garnish, you can top each dessert with a fresh or thawed frozen strawberry.

- *Blender*

3¹⁄₂ oz	frozen strawberries, halved	100 g
1	large ripe banana (see tip) or medium avocado	1
2 to 3 tbsp	Sour Cream (page 92)	30 to 45 mL
	Grated zest of ¹⁄₂ lime	
	Freeze-dried strawberries (see tip)	

1. In blender, combine frozen strawberries, banana and desired amount of sour cream; purée until smooth.

2. Spoon purée into two dessert bowls and add half the lime zest to each, stirring well. Serve garnished with freeze-dried strawberries.

Variation
Replace the strawberries with frozen sweet cherries and omit the lime zest.

Berry Iced Kefir

Makes 6 servings

Looking for a delicious way to use your homemade coconut kefir? You found it! The iced kefir is intended to have a somewhat sour taste, but you can add a little honey to sweeten it if you like.

Tip

The iced kefir can be stored in the freezer for up to 6 months.

- *Blender*
- *Electric mixer*

6 oz	frozen raspberries, strawberries or blueberries	175 g
1 tbsp	Vanilla Vodka (page 79)	15 mL
1 cup	Coconut Kefir (page 93)	250 mL
	Raw honey (optional)	

1. In blender, combine raspberries and vanilla vodka; purée until smooth.

2. Transfer raspberry purée to a bowl, add kefir and, using electric mixer, beat for 2 minutes. Taste and add a little honey, if desired.

3. Pour into an airtight container and freeze until firm, about 6 hours.

Raspberry Sorbet

Makes 4 servings

Here's a sweet, refreshing dessert that's free of any dairy.

Tips

Publisher's note: Although raw eggs are considered nourishing in the GAPS diet, they may contain salmonella (see sidebar, page 22). If you prefer to err on the side of caution, you can replace the raw egg whites in this recipe with 6 tbsp (90 mL) pasteurized liquid egg whites or simply use the whites from pasteurized in-shell eggs, if available. Note that, while pasteurized eggs are not part of the GAPS nutritional protocol, food safety must be your first priority.

In place of the Vanilla Honey, you can use regular honey and add 1 tsp (5 mL) Vanilla Vodka (page 79).

The sorbet can be stored in the freezer for up to 3 months.

- *Electric mixer*
- *Blender*
- *Ice cream maker (optional)*

3	large egg whites (see tip)	3
8 tsp	Vanilla Honey (page 78)	40 mL
8 oz	frozen raspberries, thawed slightly	250 g

1. In a large bowl, using electric mixer, beat egg whites until very stiff. Gradually add vanilla honey, whisking.
2. In blender, process raspberries until mashed.
3. Using a silicone spatula, fold mashed raspberries into egg whites.
4. Transfer to ice cream maker and freeze according to manufacturer's instructions, or pour into an airtight container and freeze until firm, about 6 hours, carefully stirring the sorbet a few times while it's freezing, if desired.

Variation

Other berries may be substituted, but if you use red currants, you'll need to add more honey. Add more than you think you should, as freezing subdues the sweetness.

Apple or Pear Clafoutis

Makes 6 servings

I got this recipe from my daughter, Karen's, American pen pal Tressa. We adjusted it slightly, and we love it! It's great for dessert or a special breakfast.

Tips

Bitter almonds are not available in all areas; if you can get them, it adds a special twist to the flavor, but if you can't buy them, simply omit it.

If using vanilla extract, check the label to make sure it contains only vanilla, water and alcohol, with no other additives.

Variation

Instead of baking in one large dish, you may choose to bake individual portions in six ⅔-cup (150 mL) individual baking dishes or ramekins for 25 to 30 minutes. These small clafoutis are well-suited for events such as a birthday breakfast.

- *Preheat oven to 340°F (170°C), with rack set in second-lowest position*
- *9-inch (23 cm) ceramic quiche dish or shallow pie plate*
- *Nut grinder (see box, page 75)*
- *Blender*

10 tsp	butter or Clarified Butter (page 68), divided	50 mL
1⅔ oz	dried soaked almonds (see page 74)	50 g
1	bitter almond, very finely chopped (optional; see tip)	1
4	large eggs	4
½ cup	Sour Cream (page 92)	125 mL
8 tsp	honey	40 mL
1 tsp	Vanilla Vodka (page 79) or pure vanilla extract	5 mL
¼ tsp	salt	1 mL
Pinch	finely grated nutmeg	Pinch
	Grated zest of ½ lemon	
3	large apples or pears, cut lengthwise into thin wedges	3
1 to 2 tsp	ground cinnamon	5 to 10 mL

1. Place 2 tsp (10 mL) butter in quiche dish; place dish in preheated oven for 2 minutes to melt butter. Use a pastry brush to coat pan evenly. Set aside. (Leave oven on.)

2. In nut grinder, grind almonds into medium-fine flour. Transfer to a large bowl and stir in bitter almond (if using).

3. In blender, combine the remaining butter, eggs, sour cream, honey, vanilla vodka, salt, nutmeg and lemon zest; process until smooth. Pour over almond flour and stir well.

4. Spread apples in quiche dish. Spread egg mixture evenly over apples. Sift cinnamon to taste over top.

5. Bake in preheated oven for 40 minutes or just until golden and puffed around the edges and set in the center. Let cool slightly and serve warm or let cool to room temperature.

Berry Clafoutis

Makes 6 servings

The original French clafoutis is a dessert cake with cherries. But berries are just as delicious when they are in season, and frozen berries can be used too. Small clafoutis (see variation) can even be added to a picnic basket.

Tips

Bitter almonds are not available in all areas; if you can get them, it adds a special twist to the flavor, but if you can't buy them, simply omit it.

For the berries, you can use whole raspberries or blueberries or halved strawberries. Or try halved pitted cherries. You need enough to cover the bottom of the pie plate in a single layer.

- **Preheat oven to 340°F (170°C), with rack set in second-lowest position**
- **9-inch (23 cm) ceramic quiche dish or shallow pie plate**
- **Nut grinder (see box, page 75)**
- **Blender**

10 tsp	butter or Clarified Butter (page 68), divided	50 mL
1$\frac{2}{3}$ oz	dried soaked almonds (see page 74)	50 g
1	bitter almond, very finely chopped (optional; see tip)	1
4	large eggs	4
$\frac{1}{2}$ cup	Sour Cream (page 92)	125 mL
3 tbsp	honey	45 mL
1 tsp	Vanilla Vodka (page 79) or pure vanilla extract	5 mL
$\frac{1}{4}$ tsp	salt	1 mL
	Grated zest of $\frac{1}{2}$ lemon	
8 oz	fresh or frozen berries (see tip)	250 g

1. Place 2 tsp (10 mL) butter in quiche dish; place dish in preheated oven for 2 minutes to melt butter. Use a pastry brush to coat pan evenly. Set aside. (Leave oven on.)

2. In nut grinder, grind almonds into medium-fine flour. Transfer to a large bowl and stir in bitter almond (if using).

3. In blender, combine the remaining butter, eggs, sour cream, honey, vanilla vodka, salt and lemon zest; process until smooth. Pour over almond flour and stir well.

4. Place berries in quiche dish. (If using halved strawberries or cherries, place them cut side down.) Spread egg mixture evenly over berries.

5. Bake in preheated oven for 35 to 40 minutes or until golden and puffed around the edges and set in the center. Let cool slightly and serve warm or let cool to room temperature.

Variation

Instead of baking in one large dish, you may choose to bake individual portions in six $\frac{2}{3}$-cup (150 mL) individual baking dishes or ramekins for 25 to 30 minutes.

Ginger Pumpkin Pie

Makes 10 to 12 servings		

With some GAPS-friendly ingredients already prepared and at hand, this pie is easy to put together. Serve it with Sour Cream (page 92), cold Coconut Whipped Cream (page 261) or a spoonful of Honey Nut Ice Cream (page 231). Start preparing the crust and filling the day before you wish to bake the pie.

Tips

For the nut flour, use a mixture of hazelnuts, walnuts and almonds.

Make sure to prepare the beans properly, as described on page 72. Keep in mind that, even after this preparation, some people may find them difficult or impossible to digest.

Choose a good-quality brand of unflavored gelatin powder made from grass-fed animals, such as Great Lakes or Vital Protein. For more information, see page 55.

- *Nut grinder (see box, page 75)*
- *Strainer lined with cheesecloth*
- *10-inch (25 cm) pie plate, buttered*

Crust

3⅔ oz	dried soaked mixed nuts (see tip and page 74)	110 g
⅓ cup	mashed cooked white beans (see page 72)	75 mL
2 tbsp + 2 tsp	fine coconut flour	20 g
1 tsp	salt	5 mL
1	large egg white, beaten	1
¼ cup	honey	60 mL
3 tbsp	Clarified Butter (page 68), melted	45 mL
	Additional fine coconut flour	
1½ tsp	unflavored gelatin powder, divided	7 mL

Pumpkin Filling

1⅔ cups	Baked Pumpkin or Squash (page 77)	400 mL
4	large eggs	4
¼ cup	Sour Cream (page 92) or coconut cream	60 mL
2 tbsp	grated gingerroot	30 mL
2 tsp	ground cinnamon	10 mL
½ tsp	ground allspice	2 mL
½ tsp	ground ginger	2 mL
Pinch	salt	Pinch
1	vanilla bean	1
8 tsp	honey	40 mL
1 oz	dried soaked pecans or walnuts (see page 74), coarsely chopped	30 g

Day 1

1. *Crust:* In nut grinder, grind nuts into medium-fine flour. Transfer to a medium bowl.

2. Add beans, coconut flour, salt, egg white, honey and clarified butter to nut flour, stirring to make a soft dough. Cover and refrigerate for 1 day.

3. *Filling:* Set lined strainer over a bowl and spoon pumpkin into strainer. Cover and refrigerate overnight to drain.

Tips

Coconut cream is the thick fatty layer that rises to the top and solidifies when coconut milk is refrigerated.

Garnish with small shapes carved from raw apple, pumpkin seeds or other GAPS-friendly cake garnishes.

Day 2

4. *Crust:* Preheat oven to 415°F (210°C), with rack set in second-lowest position.

5. Sprinkle work surface with coconut flour. Roll out three-quarters of the dough (about $7\frac{1}{2}$ oz/225 g) to fit bottom of pie plate. (The dough may be difficult to work with, but you can place smaller pieces of dough in the plate one at a time until the bottom is covered, then press pieces together to make cohesive. Note that the sides of the plate should not yet be covered.)

6. Sprinkle a fine layer of gelatin over the crust, using 1 tsp (5 mL) of the gelatin, and pat it into the dough.

7. Bake crust for 9 to 10 minutes or until starting to turn golden. Let cool. Reduce oven temperature to 350°F (180°C).

8. *Filling:* Meanwhile, in a bowl, whisk together eggs, sour cream, grated ginger, cinnamon, allspice, ground ginger and salt.

9. Split vanilla bean and stir seeds into honey. Add honey mixture and drained pumpkin to egg mixture and whisk to combine.

10. Grease cooled sides of pie plate. Divide the remaining dough into several small pieces and, on a table sprinkled with coconut flour, press each piece flat with the back of your hand. Cut the pieces to match the depth of the sides of the pie plate.

11. Sprinkle each piece of dough with a fine layer of the remaining gelatin and pat it into the dough.

12. Place one piece of dough at a time around the sides of the pie plate, with the gelatin-covered side facing out. Press the pieces firmly together and to the bottom crust. Cut off excess dough for an even edge.

13. Scatter pecans over bottom crust, then pour in pumpkin filling.

14. Bake pie for about 40 minutes or until crust is golden brown and filling is puffed around the edges and just set in the center. Watch to make sure the edges don't turn black; if crust is getting too dark before the filling is set, arrange strips of foil around the crust. Let cool completely on a wire rack. Cover loosely and refrigerate for about 1 hour, until chilled, or for up to 8 hours.

Tarte Tatin à la GAPS

Makes 6 servings

Home bakers often find it challenging to make pies and tarts for the GAPS diet that have both fantastic taste and an appealing texture. I've done all the problem-solving for you with this upside-down apple tart, though you do have to plan ahead and prepare the dough the day before. Serve with Sour Cream (page 92) or coconut butter.

Tips

To line the pan, cut a piece of parchment paper in a circle slightly larger than the bottom of the pan. Press the paper firmly to the bottom of the pan and then clamp on the ring so that only the bottom is lined. Brush the paper with a little butter.

Choose cooking apples that hold their shape when cooked, such as Braeburn, Crispin (Mutsu), Golden Delicious, Granny Smith, Honeycrisp, Jonagold or Northern Spy.

- *Nut grinder (see box, page 75)*
- *Blender*
- *Candy or instant-read thermometer*
- *8½-inch (22 cm) springform pan, bottom lined with parchment paper (see tip) and buttered*

Dough

5 oz	dried soaked almonds (see page 74), divided	150 g
⅓ cup	cold butter	75 mL
3 tbsp	honey	45 mL
½	large egg white (2 tbsp/30 mL)	½

Filling

3 tbsp	honey	45 mL
8 tsp	butter	40 mL
3	cooking apples, peeled and cut lengthwise into 12 wedges	3

Day 1

1. *Dough:* In nut grinder, grind half the almonds into fine flour; transfer to a bowl. Grind the remaining half into medium-fine flour.

2. In blender, process fine almond flour with cold butter until combined. Add medium-fine almond flour and honey; process to combine. Transfer to a medium bowl.

3. Add egg white and knead to form a dough. Wrap in plastic wrap and refrigerate for 1 day.

Day 2

4. *Filling:* In a skillet, heat honey over medium heat until it starts to caramelize and reaches about 220°F (105°C). (It happens fast, so watch that it doesn't burn.) Stir in butter, then stir in apples. Reduce heat and simmer, gently turning apples occasionally, for 20 to 30 minutes or until apples have soaked up most of the sauce and are tender.

5. Meanwhile, preheat oven to 350°F (180°C), with rack set in second-lowest position.

Tips

Be sure to let the apples cool off before covering them with dough; otherwise, the dough will become unmanageable.

Wait until the last minute before turning the tart out of the pan, so the bottom will maintain its crispness.

6. Carefully transfer apple mixture to the springform pan. Let cool completely.

7. On a piece of parchment paper, trace a circle around the bottom of the pan, then flip paper over. Place dough in middle of circle. Using your hand, pound dough flat so it fills the circle. With a long, sharp knife, loosen dough from paper. Lift dough up, along with paper, and invert on top of cooled apples so that it lands like a lid. Carefully pull off paper.

8. Bake tart for 20 minutes or until pastry is golden and firm. Let cool slightly.

9. Right before serving, invert a serving platter onto the tart, then flip both over to turn the tart out of the pan. Carefully remove parchment paper from caramelized apples.

Mince Tarts

Makes 12 tarts

In medieval England, mince tarts were made with real minced meat mixed with spices and chopped dried fruit. Today the meat is left out, but we still call the fruit filling "mincemeat." These tarts have a nice crisp crust and a spicy, caramelized flavor. They require a couple days of preparation.

Tips

For the nut flour, use a mixture of your favorite dried soaked nuts (see page 74).

Choose a good-quality brand of unflavored gelatin powder made from grass-fed animals, such as Great Lakes or Vital Protein. For more information, see page 55.

- *Nut grinder (see box, page 75)*
- *12-cup muffin pan, greased*

Mincemeat

⅔ cup	raisins or sultanas, chopped	150 mL
6	pitted medium dates, chopped	6
3	dried apricots, chopped	3
3 tbsp	dried cranberries	45 mL
2 tbsp	whisky (not smoked)	30 mL
	Grated zest and juice of ½ orange	
	Grated zest and juice of ¼ lemon	
5 tsp	Clarified Butter (page 68), melted	25 mL
½ tsp	Holiday Spice Blend (page 266)	2 mL
½ tsp	ground cinnamon	2 mL
¼ tsp	grated nutmeg	1 mL
½	apple, grated	½

Crusts

2⅔ oz	dried soaked mixed nuts (see tip)	80 g
3 tbsp	finely grated carrot	45 mL
½ tsp	salt	2 mL
⅓ cup	Clarified Butter (page 68), melted	75 mL
3 tbsp	honey	45 mL
½	large egg white (2 tbsp/30 mL)	½
1 tsp	unflavored gelatin powder	5 mL

Day 1

1. *Mincemeat:* In a bowl, combine raisins, dates, apricots, cranberries, whisky, orange zest, orange juice, lemon zest and lemon juice. Cover and let soak for 1 day.

2. *Crusts:* In nut grinder, grind nuts into fine flour. Transfer to a medium bowl.

3. Add carrot and salt to nut flour, stirring to combine. Add clarified butter and honey, stirring well. Add egg white and sprinkle in gelatin; stir well (the dough will be rather soft). Cover and refrigerate for 1 day.

Tips

The mincemeat can be prepared through step 4 and stored in an airtight container in the refrigerator for up to 5 days. If you have prepared mincemeat and dough, it is easy to finish making the tarts.

Garnish the cooled tarts with finely grated orange zest, Marzipan (page 259) or another GAPS-friendly garnish.

Day 2

4. *Mincemeat:* In a bowl, combine clarified butter, spice blend, cinnamon and nutmeg. Add to raisin mixture, along with apple, and stir well.

5. *Crusts:* Preheat oven to 400°F (200°C), with rack set in second-lowest position.

6. Cut dough into 12 equal pieces and shape into balls. Place balls in prepared muffin cups and press into bottoms and up the sides; trim off excess dough at the rim on top.

7. Bake crusts for about 13 minutes or until they become bubbly and the sides collapse (don't worry; just make sure they don't turn black). Let cool completely in pan for 30 minutes. Reduce oven temperature to 350°F (180°C).

8. Place a spoonful of mincemeat in each crust, press well and smooth the tops.

9. Bake tarts for about 8 minutes or until golden brown. Let cool in pan on a wire rack until lukewarm, then transfer tarts to rack to cool completely.

Rhubarb Crumble

Makes 6 servings

For best results, start making the dough the day before you want to bake the crumble. It is delicious served with Sour Cream (page 92), Honey Nut Ice Cream (page 231) or Coconut Whipped Cream (page 261).

Tips

You can replace the vanilla bean with 2 tsp (10 mL) Vanilla Vodka (page 79) or pure vanilla extract.

Placing the dough in the refrigerator overnight will firm it up and make it easier to crumble, but if you'd prefer to make the dessert all in one day, just spread the dough on the fruit with a spoon or knife instead of crumbling it. With this method, start the recipe by preparing the filling, to let the rhubarb marinate a little while you make the dough.

The crumble is best when served warm, and it is crispiest right after it comes out of the oven.

- **Nut grinder (see box, page 75)**
- **6-cup (1.5 L) baking dish, greased**

Dough

5 oz	dried soaked almonds (see page 74), divided	150 g
1 tbsp	honey	15 mL
1/4 cup	butter or Clarified Butter (page 68)	60 mL

Filling

2/3 cup	honey	150 mL
1/2	vanilla bean, split	1/2
	Grated zest and juice of 1/4 lemon	
1 lb	rhubarb stalks (without leaves), cut into 3/4-inch (2 cm) pieces	500 g

Day 1

1. *Dough:* In nut grinder, grind 3 oz (90 g) of the almonds into fine flour and transfer to a small bowl. Finely chop the remaining almonds and add to almond flour.

2. In a small saucepan, melt honey over low heat. Remove from heat and stir in butter until melted.

3. Pour honey mixture into almond flour and knead well. Cover bowl with a plate and refrigerate overnight (see tip).

4. *Filling:* In a medium bowl, stir together honey, vanilla bean, lemon zest and lemon juice.

5. Fold in rhubarb until evenly coated. Cover and let stand on counter overnight.

Day 2

6. Preheat oven to 350°F (180°C), with rack set in second-lowest position. Remove vanilla bean, pour rhubarb mixture into prepared baking dish and crumble dough on top.

7. Bake for 25 to 30 minutes or until rhubarb is tender and topping is golden and crisp.

Variation

Apple Crumble: In place of the rhubarb filling, combine 4 cooking apples, peeled and coarsely chopped, with 2 tsp (10 mL) ground cinnamon. Transfer to prepared baking dish, sprinkle with a handful of raisins and crumble dough on top. Bake as directed.

Banana Mazarin Cake

Makes 8 servings

Coconut Whipped Cream (page 261) tastes wonderful with this classic Danish cake, as do fresh strawberries, raspberries and blueberries.

Tips

If you wish to bake a flan without nuts, you can omit the walnuts.

If using vanilla extract, check the label to make sure it contains only vanilla, water and alcohol, with no other additives.

- **Preheat oven to 275°F (135°C), with rack set in second-lowest position**
- **Nut grinder (see box, page 75)**
- **Blender**
- **9-inch (23 cm) glass or ceramic tart dish, greased**

1²⁄₃ oz	dried soaked walnuts (see page 74), divided	50 g
3	ripe bananas	3
5	large eggs	5
½ cup	butter	125 mL
3 tbsp	honey	45 mL
1 tsp	Vanilla Vodka (page 79) or pure vanilla extract	5 mL

1. In nut grinder, grind half the walnuts into medium-fine flour; transfer to a medium bowl. Finely chop the remaining walnuts and add to nut flour.

2. In blender, combine bananas, eggs, butter, honey and vanilla vodka; blend until smooth. Pour over walnut flour mixture and stir to combine. Pour into prepared dish.

3. Bake in preheated oven for about 80 minutes or until light golden brown.

Variation

Instead of a tart dish, you can use six ²⁄₃-cup (150 mL) individual ramekins and bake for 60 minutes.

Coconut Cake

Makes 6 to
8 servings

*This cake can be eaten as is
or used as a base for fruit,
Coconut Whipped Cream
(page 261) or Sour Cream
(page 92). Or make one
of the variations.*

Tips

If using vanilla extract, check
the label to make sure it
contains only vanilla, water
and alcohol, with no other
additives.

Although raw honey is
recommended on the
GAPS diet, its nutrients
are destroyed by heat, so
save it for recipes that are
not heated and use regular
honey in baking and cooking.

- *Preheat oven to 340°F (170°C), with rack set in second-lowest position*
- *Electric mixer*
- *10-inch (25 cm) springform pan, brushed with coconut oil*

4	large egg yolks	4
1/4 cup	honey	60 mL
1 1/4 cups	unsweetened shredded coconut	300 mL
2 tsp	Vanilla Vodka (page 79) or pure vanilla extract	10 mL
5	large egg whites	5
2 tsp	honey	10 mL

1. In a medium bowl, using electric mixer, beat egg yolks and 1/4 cup (60 mL) honey until pale and thickened. Beat in coconut and vanilla vodka.

2. In a medium bowl, using clean beaters, beat egg whites until medium stiff. Drizzle in 2 tsp (10 mL) honey for stabilization and beat until very stiff peaks form.

3. Using a silicone spatula, gently fold one-quarter of the egg whites into egg yolk mixture until there are no more "islands" of whites in the dough. Repeat with another quarter, then the remaining egg whites. Spread batter in prepared pan.

4. Bake in preheated oven for 25 minutes or until golden and puffed around the edges and set in the center. Remove cake from pan and let cool completely on a wire rack.

Variations

Orange Coconut Cake: When cake has cooled to lukewarm, pour 2/3 cup (150 mL) Orange Sauce (page 266) over top and let it soak into the cake while it is cooling completely. Using a paring knife, peel an orange, including the white membrane. Cut orange flesh into ultra-thin slices and use to garnish the cake.

Coconut Lemon Moon Cake: Cut cake in half vertically and place half on a platter. Spread 1/2 cup (125 mL) Lemon Buttercream (page 262) over cake and top with the other cake half. Spread a thin layer of buttercream on top. Decorate cake with grated lemon zest.

Coconut Mocha Moon Cake: Cut cake in half vertically and place half on a platter. Spread 1/2 cup (125 mL) Mocha Buttercream (page 263) over cake and top with the other cake half. Spread a thin layer of buttercream on top. Garnish cake with whole coffee beans (not to be eaten!) or Hazelnut Croquant made with coffee (page 267).

Coconut Cake with Apple and Almond Croquant: When cake has cooled completely, cover with 1 2/3 cups (400 mL) cold Applesauce (page 219) and sprinkle Almond Croquant (variation, page 267) on top. Serve immediately.

Carrot Coconut Cupcakes

Makes 6 cupcakes

These moist, yummy cupcakes are free of milk products, flour, eggs, nuts and nightshades.

Tip

If using vanilla extract, check the label to make sure it contains only vanilla, water and alcohol, with no other additives.

- *Preheat oven to 400°F (200°C), with rack set in second-lowest position*
- *12-cup muffin pan, 6 cups greased with coconut oil*

4 tsp	coconut oil, melted	20 mL
2 tsp	Vanilla Vodka (page 79) or pure vanilla extract	10 mL
1 tsp	honey	5 mL
Pinch	salt	Pinch
2/3 cup	finely grated carrots (3 1/2 oz/100 g)	150 mL
1/3 cup	unsweetened shredded coconut	75 mL
1/4 cup	raisins	60 mL
	Cold Coconut Whipped Cream (page 261)	
	Thin lime slices	

1. In a medium bowl, whisk together coconut oil, vanilla vodka, honey and salt, stirring to dissolve honey and salt. Add carrots, coconut and raisins, stirring until evenly moistened.

2. Divide batter evenly among prepared muffin cups.

3. Bake in preheated oven for 20 minutes or until golden brown. Let cool in pan on a wire rack for 5 minutes, then transfer cupcakes to rack to cool completely.

4. Serve topped with coconut whipped cream and lime slices.

Christmas Puddings

Makes 14 to 18 cakes

These Christmas puddings are particularly delicious when freshly baked, but they will retain their chewy and caramel consistency for several days.

Tips

When done, these cakes should be dark but not black! Keep an eye on them; you may need to turn down the heat during baking.

Top the cakes with Lemon Buttercream (page 262) or Bourbon Butter (page 264) and garnish with Marzipan (page 259), finely chopped dried cranberries, fresh or dried orange slices or any other sugar-free garnish.

Although these are best freshly baked, you can store the cooled cakes in an airtight container at room temperature for up to 3 days or in the refrigerator for up to 1 week.

- *Nut grinder (see box, page 75)*
- *Two 12-cup muffin pans, 14 to 18 cups buttered*

8 oz	dried dates, pitted and chopped	250 g
7 oz	raisins or sultanas	200 g
1 oz	unsweetened dried cranberries	30 g
	Finely grated zest and juice of 1 orange	
	Finely grated zest and juice of 1/2 lemon	
1/4 cup	whisky (not smoked) or brandy	60 mL
3 oz	dried soaked almonds (see page 74)	90 g
1/2 cup	butter or Clarified Butter (page 68), melted	125 mL
1/4 cup	honey	60 mL
1 1/2 tsp	Holiday Spice Blend (page 266)	7 mL
1 1/2 tsp	ground cinnamon	7 mL
2	large eggs, beaten	2
1	carrot (1 2/3 oz/50 g), peeled and finely grated	1
7 oz	dried soaked walnuts or pecans, coarsely chopped	200 g
1/2 cup	Baked Pumpkin or Squash (page 77), mashed	125 mL

Day 1

1. In a medium bowl, combine dates, raisins, cranberries, orange zest, orange juice, lemon zest, lemon juice and whisky. Cover and let soak for 1 day, stirring occasionally.

Day 2

2. Preheat oven to 300°F (150°C), with rack set in second-lowest position.

3. In nut grinder, grind almonds into fine flour.

4. In a small bowl, stir together butter, honey, spice blend and cinnamon.

5. Add almond flour, butter mixture, eggs, carrot, walnuts and pumpkin to soaked fruit, stirring until evenly blended.

6. Divide batter evenly among prepared muffin cups (they will only rise slightly).

7. Bake for 70 to 80 minutes or until well browned. Let cool in pans on a wire rack for 15 minutes, then transfer cakes to rack to cool completely.

Blueberry Muffins

Makes 15 muffins

These are good as part of a brunch, as a snack on the go, or for a birthday breakfast. Serve them as is, with Sour Cream (page 92) or with Coconut Whipped Cream (page 261).

Tips

If using vanilla extract, check the label to make sure it contains only vanilla, water and alcohol, with no other additives.

The cooled muffins can be stored in an airtight container at room temperature for up to 3 days, in the refrigerator for up to 1 week or in the freezer for up to 1 year. If frozen, let thaw at room temperature for 1 to 2 hours before serving.

- **Preheat oven to 340°F (170°C), with rack set in second-lowest position**
- **Nut grinder (see box, page 75)**
- **Blender**
- **Electric mixer**
- **Two 12-cup muffin pans, 15 cups greased**

5 oz	dried soaked hazelnuts (see page 74)	150 g
1/3 cup	unsweetened shredded coconut	75 mL
1/4 tsp	salt	1 mL
2	ripe bananas	2
1	large egg yolk	1
	Grated zest of 1/2 orange	
1/3 cup	honey	75 mL
8 tsp	butter, Clarified Butter (page 68) or coconut oil	40 mL
1 tsp	Vanilla Vodka (page 79) or pure vanilla extract	5 mL
3	large egg whites	3
2 2/3 oz	frozen blueberries, thawed	80 g

1. In nut grinder, grind hazelnuts into medium-fine flour. Transfer to a large bowl.

2. Add coconut and salt to nut flour, stirring to combine.

3. In blender, combine bananas, egg yolk, orange zest, honey, butter and vanilla vodka; blend until smooth. Pour over flour mixture and stir just until evenly moistened.

4. In a small bowl, using electric mixer, beat egg whites until stiff. Using a silicone spatula, gently fold one-quarter of the egg whites into batter until no "islands" of egg white are left. Repeat with another quarter, then the remaining egg whites.

5. Spoon enough batter into prepared muffin cups so they are filled halfway. Place 1 tsp (5 mL) blueberries in each cup, followed by another 1 tsp (5 mL) batter. With a fork, stir each muffin a little so that blueberries are visible.

6. Bake in preheated oven for about 25 minutes or until lightly browned. Let cool in pans on a wire rack for 10 minutes, then transfer muffins to rack to cool completely.

Cocoa and Raspberry Muffins

Makes 15 muffins

Raw cacao is not the first thing to eat when you start the GAPS diet. But when your health has improved, you might feel like trying these nice muffins.

Tips

You can use pure vanilla extract in place of the vanilla vodka, but check the label to make sure it contains only vanilla, water and alcohol, with no other additives.

If you can't find freeze-dried raspberries, you can use fresh or thawed frozen raspberries for the garnish.

The muffins can be prepared through step 6, then stored in an airtight container at room temperature for up to 3 days, in the refrigerator for up to 1 week or in the freezer for up to 1 year. If frozen, let thaw at room temperature for 1 to 2 hours. Frost and garnish just before serving.

- Preheat oven to 340°F (170°C), with rack set in second-lowest position
- Nut grinder (see box, page 75)
- Blender
- Electric mixer
- Two 12-cup muffin pans, 15 cups greased

8 1/3 oz	dried soaked almonds (see page 74)	260 g
1/3 cup	unsweetened cocoa powder	75 mL
2 tbsp	unsweetened shredded coconut	30 mL
1 1/2 tbsp	chopped raw cacao nibs	22 mL
1/4 tsp	salt	1 mL
3	ripe bananas	3
6 tbsp	honey	90 mL
5 tsp	butter, Clarified Butter (page 68) or coconut oil	25 mL
2 tsp	Vanilla Vodka (page 79)	10 mL
3	large egg whites	3
30	frozen raspberries, separated	30
1/2 cup	Lemon Buttercream (page 262)	125 mL
	Freeze-dried raspberries (see tip)	

1. In nut grinder, grind almonds into medium-fine flour. Transfer to a large bowl.

2. Sift cocoa powder into almond flour. Stir in coconut, cacao nibs and salt.

3. In blender, combine bananas, honey, butter and vanilla vodka; blend until smooth. Pour over flour mixture and stir just until evenly moistened.

4. In a small bowl, using electric mixer, beat egg whites until stiff. Using a silicone spatula, gently fold one-quarter of the egg whites into batter until no "islands" of egg white are left. Repeat with another quarter, then the remaining egg whites.

5. Place 2 frozen raspberries in each prepared muffin cup. Divide batter evenly among cups.

6. Bake in preheated oven for about 25 minutes or until golden brown. Let cool in pans on a wire rack for 10 minutes, then transfer muffins to rack to cool completely.

7. Using a knife with a wide blade that has been rinsed in hot water, spread buttercream in a thin layer over muffins. Garnish with freeze-dried raspberries.

Pear Walnut Muffins

Makes 14 muffins

Whether you eat them at home or bring them with you on the go, muffins like these are really good alternatives to floury, sugary cakes and cookies. When you get the hang of baking this way, you can create your own favorite muffins with the fruit filling you prefer.

Tips

This recipe contains pulp from juicing. When you're planning to use the pulp from juicing, the vegetables must be peeled and clean before you juice them.

If using vanilla extract, check the label to make sure it contains only vanilla, water and alcohol, with no other additives.

The cooled muffins can be stored in an airtight container at room temperature for up to 3 days, in the refrigerator for up to 1 week or in the freezer for up to 1 year. If frozen, let thaw at room temperature for 1 to 2 hours before serving.

- *Preheat oven to 340°F (170°C), with rack set in second-lowest position*
- *Nut grinder (see box, page 75)*
- *Blender*
- *Two 12-cup muffin pans, 14 cups greased*

1²/₃ oz	dried soaked almonds (see page 74)	50 g
1²/₃ oz	pulp from juiced carrot, apple or pear (see tip)	50 g
6 tbsp	unsweetened shredded coconut	90 mL
¼ tsp	salt	1 mL
4	large eggs, separated	4
8 tsp	honey	40 mL
1 tsp	Vanilla Vodka (page 79) or pure vanilla extract	5 mL
2	medium-large ripe pears, peeled and diced	2
1 oz	dried soaked walnuts (see page 74), coarsely chopped	30 g
1 tbsp	raw cacao nibs	15 mL
14	dried soaked walnut halves	14

1. In nut grinder, grind almonds into medium-fine flour. Transfer to a large bowl.

2. In blender, combine pulp, coconut and salt; blend until it no longer lumps together. Pour over flour and stir until combined.

3. In a small bowl, using electric mixer, beat egg yolks and honey until pale and thickened. Beat in vanilla vodka. Pour over flour mixture and stir just until evenly moistened. Fold in pears, chopped walnuts and cacao nibs.

4. In a medium bowl, using clean beaters, beat 3 egg whites until very stiff. Using a silicone spatula, gently fold one-quarter of the egg whites into batter until no "islands" of egg white are left. Repeat with another quarter, then the remaining egg whites.

5. Divide batter evenly among prepared muffin cups and top each with a walnut half.

6. Bake in preheated oven for 20 to 25 minutes or until golden brown. Let cool in pan on a wire rack for 10 minutes, then transfer muffins to rack to cool completely.

Honey Cookies

Makes 24 cookies

Honey cookies taste great spread with butter. They're a great choice when you're baking for the holidays, but may be enjoyed all year round.

Tips

You can use Clarified Butter (page 68) in place of butter, but add a pinch of salt to the flour mixture in that case.

As with most other GAPS-friendly cakes and cookies, these are best freshly baked, but you can store the cooled cookies in an airtight container at room temperature for up to 1 week. Since the cookies do not contain starchy flour, they tend to quickly turn soft. You can resurrect their crispness by placing them in a 150°F (65°C) dehydrator or oven with the rack set in the middle position for 15 to 20 minutes.

- *Blender*
- *Baking sheet, greased*

⅔ cup	coconut flour	150 mL
2 tsp	ground cinnamon	10 mL
¼ tsp	ground cloves	1 mL
	Finely grated zest of 1 orange	
3 tbsp	honey	45 mL
⅓ cup	butter (see tip), melted	75 mL

1. In blender, combine coconut flour, cinnamon, cloves, orange zest and honey; blend until combined. Add butter and blend until a smooth dough forms.

2. Transfer dough to a bowl, cover and refrigerate for 1 hour.

3. Preheat oven to 340°F (170°C), with rack set in middle position.

4. Divide dough into 3 equal portions, then divide each portion into 8 equal pieces. Roll each piece into a ball and place on prepared baking sheet, spacing them about 1 inch (2.5 cm) apart. With the palm of your hand, press flat to about 1½ inches (4 cm) in diameter. (If you want the cookies to be nicely rounded, use a round cookie cutter to trim the edges.)

5. Bake for 8 minutes or until golden. Let cool on pan on a wire rack for 5 minutes, then transfer cookies to rack to cool completely.

Variation

Ginger Cookies: Substitute 2 tsp (10 mL) ground ginger for the cinnamon, cloves and orange zest.

Coconut Cookies

Makes 24 cookies

These cookies resemble biscuits and taste especially great with blue cheese.

Tips

You can use Clarified Butter (page 68) in place of butter, but add a pinch of salt to the flour mixture in that case.

As with most other GAPS-friendly cakes and cookies, these are best freshly baked, but you can store the cooled cookies in an airtight container at room temperature for up to 1 week. Since the cookies do not contain starchy flour, they tend to quickly turn soft. You can resurrect their crispness by placing them in a 150°F (65°C) dehydrator or oven with the rack set in the middle position for 15 to 20 minutes.

- *Blender*
- *Large baking sheet, greased*

²⁄₃ cup	coconut flour	150 mL
¹⁄₃ cup	butter (see tip), melted	75 mL
3 tbsp	honey	45 mL

1. In blender, combine coconut flour, butter and honey; blend until a smooth dough forms.

2. Transfer dough to a bowl, cover and refrigerate for 1 hour.

3. Preheat oven to 340°F (170°C), with rack set in middle position.

4. Divide dough into 3 equal portions, then divide each portion into 8 equal pieces. Roll each piece into a ball and place on prepared baking sheet, spacing them about 1 inch (2.5 cm) apart. With the palm of your hand, press flat to about 1¹⁄₂ inches (4 cm) in diameter. (If you want the cookies to be nicely rounded, use a round cookie cutter to trim the edges.)

5. Bake for 8 minutes or until light golden. Let cool on pan on a wire rack for 5 minutes, then transfer cookies to rack to cool completely.

Almond Tuiles

<table>
<tr><td>Makes 12 to
14 cookies</td></tr>
</table>

For a crispy contrast, serve almond tuiles as an accompaniment to ice cream, mousse, fruit jelly or another soft dessert.

Tip

As with most other GAPS-friendly cakes and cookies, these are best freshly baked, but you can store the cooled cookies in a cookie tin at room temperature for up to 1 week. Since the cookies do not contain starchy flour, they tend to quickly turn soft. You can resurrect their crispness by placing them in a 150°F (65°C) dehydrator or oven with the rack set in the middle position for 15 to 20 minutes.

- *Nut grinder (see box, page 75)*
- *Baking sheet, greased*

1⅓ oz	dried soaked almonds (see page 74)	40 g
1	large egg white	1
2 tbsp	honey	30 mL
	Finely grated zest of ½ lemon	

1. In nut grinder, grind almonds into fine flour.

2. In a medium bowl, whisk egg white and honey until honey is completely dissolved. Whisk in almond flour and lemon zest. Let dough rest for 20 minutes.

3. Meanwhile, preheat oven to 260°F (130°C), with rack set in second-lowest position.

4. Drop dough by teaspoonfuls (5 mL) on prepared baking sheet, spacing them apart. Using the back of a spoon, shape each dollop of dough into a large, very thin oval.

5. Bake for 18 to 20 minutes or until golden, with the edges slightly darker than the center. Let cool on pan for 2 minutes, then carefully lift cookies off pan and transfer to a wire rack to cool completely.

Florentines with Buttercream

Makes 12 sandwich cookies

If you feel like something quite sweet and very crispy, creamy and satisfying, these florentines are just the thing.

Tips

Experience has taught me that crisp cookies containing honey are easier to bake during the cooler months. The high humidity of summer causes them to become soft. But don't let that deter you. If they don't turn out crisp, you can dry them in a 140°F (60°C) oven or dehydrator for a couple of hours. Or you can shape them into small balls (after baking) and they turn into delicious pieces of candy (without buttercream).

If you prepare a double portion of dough, planning to bake half later, it does dry up a bit; soften it with more egg so that the cookies will flatten out while baking.

The cookies can be prepared through step 5 and stored in an airtight container at room temperature for up to 1 week. If they turn soft, crisp them as described above. Sandwich them with buttercream just before serving.

- *Preheat oven to 300°F (150°C)*
- *Nut grinder (see box, page 75)*
- *Baking sheets, lined with parchment paper*

3⅓ oz	dried soaked hazelnuts (see page 74)	110 g
⅔ cup	honey	150 mL
2 tbsp	butter, melted	30 mL
2 tsp	Vanilla Vodka (page 79) or pure vanilla extract	10 mL
⅓ cup	raisins	75 mL
6 tbsp	unsweetened shredded coconut	90 mL
1⅔ oz	dried soaked walnuts, coarsely chopped	50 g
1	large egg, beaten	1
1 cup	cold Mocha Buttercream (page 263) or Lemon Buttercream (page 262)	250 mL

1. In nut grinder, grind hazelnuts into medium-fine flour.

2. In a bowl, whisk together honey, butter and vanilla vodka. Add hazelnut flour, raisins, coconut and walnuts, stirring to combine. Fold in half of the beaten egg. The dough should be soft but not runny. You may have to use a little more egg, or even the rest of it, to get the right consistency.

3. First make a trial cookie on a prepared baking sheet to see if dough is soft enough to spread and become flat. Using two spoons, drop a walnut-size dollop of dough on prepared baking sheet. Bake in preheated oven for 14 minutes. If it does not spread, stir more egg into the dough, a little at a time, until it softens. Bake another test cookie if you're not sure.

4. Once dough is the right consistency, drop the remaining dough in walnut-size dollops on prepared baking sheets, spacing them at least 4 inches (10 cm) apart.

5. Bake one sheet at a time for 14 to 16 minutes or until golden brown. Slide parchment paper with cookies onto a wire rack and let cool. When cooled and crisp, use a palette knife to gently loosen cookies from paper.

6. Spread buttercream over half the cookies and sandwich with the remaining cookies.

Archipelago Macaroons

Makes 18 macaroons

The legendary French pastry chef Gaston Le Nôtre called his coconut macaroons "Congolesian Cliffs." In tribute, I named these cookies after the Swedish archipelagos that are near my home in Copenhagen. The cookies are easy to transport, so tuck them into your bag when you're on the go.

Tips

If using vanilla extract, check the label to make sure it contains only vanilla, water and alcohol, with no other additives.

The dough should have a consistency that allows it to be easily formed into a cone shape.

The cooled cookies can be stored in an airtight container at room temperature for up to 3 days, in the refrigerator for up to 1 week or in the freezer for up to 1 year.

- *Nut grinder (see box, page 75)*
- *Blender*
- *2 baking sheets, greased*

$4\frac{2}{3}$ oz	dried soaked hazelnuts (see page 74), divided	145 g
$1\frac{1}{2}$ to 2	large egg whites	$1\frac{1}{2}$ to 2
$\frac{1}{4}$ cup	honey	60 mL
3 tbsp	coconut oil	45 mL
1 tsp	Vanilla Vodka (page 79) or pure vanilla extract	5 mL
2 tsp	ground cinnamon	10 mL
Pinch	salt	Pinch
7 tbsp	unsweetened shredded coconut	105 mL
$\frac{1}{4}$ cup	raisins	60 mL
$2\frac{1}{2}$ tbsp	raw cacao nibs (optional)	37 mL

1. In nut grinder, grind 4 oz (125 g) hazelnuts into fine flour; transfer to a medium bowl. Coarsely chop the remaining hazelnuts and add to nut flour.

2. In blender, combine $1\frac{1}{2}$ egg whites (3 tbsp/45 mL), honey, coconut oil, vanilla vodka, cinnamon and salt; blend until smooth. Pour over nut mixture.

3. Add coconut, raisins and cocoa nibs (if using) to nut mixture and stir until evenly moistened (see tip). Let dough rest for 10 minutes.

4. Meanwhile, preheat oven to 350°F (180°C), with rack set in second-lowest position.

5. If dough seems too stiff and solid, stir in remaining $\frac{1}{2}$ egg white (1 tbsp/15 mL), but be sure it doesn't get too soft.

6. Scoop about 1 tbsp (15 mL) dough for each cookie and place on prepared baking sheets, then, using your fingers, form into an inverted cone shape. Space the cones at least 1 inch (2.5 cm) apart.

7. Bake one sheet at a time for 10 to 12 minutes or until firm around the edges and lightly browned. Let cool on pans on a wire rack for 5 minutes, then transfer to racks to cool completely.

Raspberry Coconut Macaroons

Makes 12 macaroons

When served freshly baked, these cookies are crunchy on the outside and soft on the inside.

Tips

Choose a good-quality brand of unflavored gelatin powder made from grass-fed animals, such as Great Lakes or Vital Protein. For more information, see page 55.

If you have a double boiler, this is a good time to bring it into action.

These cookies are best the same day they are baked.

- *Preheat oven to 330°F (165°C), with rack set in second-lowest position*
- *Candy or instant-read thermometer*
- *Baking sheet, greased*

1	large egg white	1
2 tbsp	liquid honey	30 mL
14 tbsp	unsweetened shredded coconut	210 mL
1/4 cup	fresh or frozen raspberries, lightly crushed	60 mL
1 tsp	unflavored gelatin powder	5 mL

1. In a medium heatproof bowl, whisk together egg white and honey. Set over a saucepan of simmering water and cook, whisking, until mixture is airy and foamy and reaches about 113°F (45°C).

2. Remove bowl from heat and stir in coconut and berries. Sprinkle with gelatin and stir thoroughly and quickly.

3. Scoop about 1 tbsp (15 mL) dough for each cookie and place on prepared baking sheet, then, using your fingers, form into an inverted cone shape. Space the cones at least 1 inch (2.5 cm) apart.

4. Bake in preheated oven for 20 minutes or until lightly browned. Let cool completely on pan on a wire rack.

New Year's Bombs

Makes 16 cookies

As with most other GAPS-friendly baked goods, these festive cookies are best freshly made, but they keep for several days. If you have kids, let them help make these! They're great for any special event, not just New Year's Eve.

Tips

The marzipan is harder and less manageable than one made with sugar, but don't give up!

Dried blueberries can be bought in large supermarkets, bulk food stores and online.

Although these are best freshly baked, you can store the cooled cookies in an airtight container, with parchment paper between layers, for up to 2 weeks in the refrigerator or up to 9 months in the freezer. If frozen, let thaw at room temperature for 1 to 2 hours before serving.

- *Preheat oven to 350°F (180°C), with rack set in second-lowest position*
- *Blender*

9 tbsp	unsweetened shredded coconut	125 mL
6 oz	Marzipan (page 259)	175 g
3	large egg whites, divided	3
1 tsp	finely grated orange zest	5 mL
1½ tbsp	dried blueberries, chopped	22 mL
4	dried soaked hazelnuts (see page 74)	4
4	dried soaked walnut halves	4

1. In blender, process coconut on high speed to a coarse powder. Add marzipan and pulse until crumbled. Transfer to a medium bowl.

2. Add 2 egg whites and knead until a soft and malleable dough forms. Divide into equal 4 portions.

3. Set aside some of the orange zest for garnish. Knead the remaining zest into 1 dough portion until incorporated. Divide that portion into 4 equal pieces and roll into balls. Place balls on a baking sheet, spacing them apart, and flatten slightly.

4. In a small bowl, lightly whisk remaining egg white. Brush over flattened orange balls and garnish with reserved orange zest.

5. Set aside some of the blueberries for garnish. Knead the remaining blueberries into another dough portion. Divide into 4 equal pieces and roll into balls. Place balls on baking sheet, spacing them apart, and flatten slightly. Brush with egg white and garnish with reserved blueberries.

6. Divide each remaining portion of dough into 4 equal pieces and roll into balls. Place on baking sheet, spacing them apart, and flatten slightly. Brush with egg white. Garnish 4 balls with a hazelnut and 4 with a walnut half.

7. Bake in preheated oven for 13 to 15 minutes or until light golden. Let cool on pan on a wire rack until firm.

Ginger Drops

Makes 28 drops

Grab a ginger drop directly from the freezer whenever you need to stabilize your blood sugar. If you want to carry them with you, use a cooler.

Tip

In recipes that are not heated, use raw honey for its added health benefits.

¼ cup	coconut oil, at room temperature	60 mL
¼ cup	raw honey	60 mL
¾ tsp	grated gingerroot	3 mL

1. In a bowl, using a fork, mash coconut oil and honey into a smooth paste (there should not be any lumps of oil). Stir in ginger.

2. Spoon 28 small dollops onto a freezer-safe plate, wrap and freeze until firm. Store in freezer for up to 1 year.

Whisky Balls

Makes 36 candies

Sugar-free, pure spirits like whisky are fine occasionally, and in modest amounts, when you are on the full GAPS diet, and the tiny amount in these candies definitely adds to the taste.

Tips

Whisky is a broad concept. A type that hasn't been smoked is the best choice for these candies.

Store in an airtight container in a cool place for up to 1 week.

- *Nut grinder (see box, page 75)*
- *Blender*

1⅔ oz	dried soaked almonds (see page 74)	50 g
8 oz	dates, pitted	250 g
	Grated zest of 1 orange	
2 tbsp	coconut oil, melted	30 mL
1 tbsp	whisky (not smoked)	15 mL
	Unsweetened shredded coconut	

1. In nut grinder, grind almonds into fine flour.

2. In a dry skillet, lightly toast almond flour over medium-low heat, stirring constantly, for about 5 minutes or until golden and fragrant. Immediately transfer to a bowl and let cool.

3. In blender, combine almond flour, dates, orange zest, coconut oil and whisky; blend until smooth.

4. Shape mixture into 36 balls, each the size of a large cherry.

5. Spread coconut in a shallow dish. Roll balls in coconut, coating evenly.

Date and Nut Balls

Makes 36 candies

Just one or two of these candies will likely satisfy your craving for sweets — but don't eat them unless you're on the full diet!

Tips

Substitute another type of nuts, such as hazelnuts, for the almonds. Don't forget to soak and dry them first.

Store in an airtight container in a cool place for up to 1 week.

- *Nut grinder (see box, page 75)*
- *High-powered blender or food processor*

1²⁄₃ oz	dried soaked almonds (see page 74)	50 g
8 oz	dates, pitted	250 g
	Grated zest of 1 orange	
2 tbsp	coconut oil, melted	30 mL

Garnish

2 to 3 tbsp	unsweetened shredded coconut	30 to 45 mL
2 tbsp	crumbled freeze-dried raspberries	30 mL
2 tbsp	unsweetened cocoa powder	30 mL

1. In nut grinder, grind almonds into fine flour.

2. In a dry skillet, lightly toast almond flour over medium-low heat, stirring constantly, for about 5 minutes or until golden and fragrant. Immediately transfer to a bowl and let cool.

3. In blender, combine almond flour, dates, orange zest and coconut oil; blend until smooth.

4. Shape mixture into 36 balls, each the size of a large cherry.

5. *Garnish:* Roll 12 balls in coconut, 12 in raspberries and 12 in cocoa (or as you please).

Marzipan

Makes about 10 oz (300 g)

You can use this marzipan as an ingredient in New Year's Bombs (page 256) or as decoration for cakes, such as Christmas Puddings (page 246). You can also roll small chunks in unsweetened shredded coconut, grated orange zest or unsweetened cocoa powder, and you'll have a sweet without additives, starch or sugar.

Tips

Bitter almonds are not available in all areas; if you can get them, they add a special twist to the flavor, but if you can't buy them, simply omit them.

Store marzipan in the refrigerator for up to 1 month or in the freezer for up to 9 months.

• *Nut grinder (see box, page 75)*

7 oz	dried blanched soaked almonds (see page 74)	200 g
3	bitter almonds (optional; see tip) Boiling water	3
6 tbsp	raw honey	90 mL

1. In nut grinder, grind dried blanched soaked almonds into fine flour.

2. In a dry skillet, lightly toast almond flour over medium-low heat, stirring constantly, for about 5 minutes or until golden and fragrant. Immediately transfer to a bowl and let cool.

3. Place bitter almonds in a bowl and pour in boiling water to scald them. Let soak until cool enough to handle, then drain and peel off skins. Chop very finely and stir into almond flour.

4. Add honey to almond mixture and knead until the mixture forms a solid mass. Shape into an elongated roll, wrap and refrigerate for at least 2 hours before use.

Walnut Fudge

Makes 24 pieces

This fudge is very popular
— even with people who
are not on the GAPS diet!
Eat it as candy or as part
of a dessert. For example,
soak some finely chopped
orange chunks in a bit of
Vanilla Vodka (page 79),
add a scoop of Honey Nut
Ice Cream (page 231) and
sprinkle with pieces of
fudge. Yum!

Tips

In recipes that are not
heated, use raw honey for
its added health benefits.

If using vanilla extract, check
the label to make sure it
contains only vanilla, water
and alcohol, with no other
additives.

The fudge will taste even
better if stored for a few days
(or weeks) in the refrigerator
or freezer.

- *Blender*
- *6½- by 4-inch (16 by 10 cm) or 9- by 3-inch (23 by 7.5 cm)
  food storage container with a tight-fitting lid, lined with
  parchment paper*

3½ oz	dried soaked walnuts (see page 74), divided	100 g
7 tbsp	unsweetened cocoa powder	105 mL
Pinch	salt	Pinch
⅓ cup	raw honey	75 mL
1 tsp	Vanilla Vodka (page 79) or pure vanilla extract	5 mL
⅓ cup	coconut oil, melted and warm	75 mL

1. Finely chop half the walnuts and coarsely chop the
   other half.

2. In blender, combine cocoa, salt, honey and vanilla vodka.
   Add warm coconut oil and blend to a smooth paste.

3. Transfer cocoa mixture to a medium bowl and fold in
   finely chopped walnuts. Pour into prepared container,
   sprinkle with coarsely chopped walnuts and press them
   into the fudge.

4. Freeze for about 3 hours or until firm. Cut into whatever
   shapes you prefer (24 pieces is just a suggestion).

Variations

Orange Fudge: Add the finely grated zest of 1 orange
in step 3 with the finely chopped walnuts.

Whisky Fudge: Add 2 tsp (10 mL) whisky (not
smoked) in step 3 with the finely chopped walnuts.

Coconut Whipped Cream

**Makes about
½ cup (125 mL)**

*Here's a really good
alternative to whipped
cream! It's delicious with
Banana Mazarin Cake
(page 243), Coconut Cake
(page 244) or Blueberry
Muffins (page 247).*

Tips

Leftover coconut cream can
be used in a smoothie.

Reserve the thin, liquid part
of the coconut milk in the
refrigerator for up to 5 days.
Use it in Thai-Style Chicken
Legs (page 153) or in a
smoothie.

In place of the vanilla seeds,
you can use ½ tsp (2 mL)
Vanilla Vodka (page 79) or
pure vanilla extract.

- *Electric mixer*

1¼ cups	cold Coconut Milk (page 76)	300 mL
¼	vanilla bean, seeds scraped	¼
Dash	raw honey	Dash

1. The cold coconut milk should have divided into two parts
   with different consistencies, a solid part on top of a liquid
   part. Carefully scoop the thick, solid cream into a cold
   bowl. Reserve the thin liquid for another use.

2. Using the electric mixer, beat cream for 1 to 2 minutes
   or until light and airy. Beat in vanilla seeds and honey.
   Use immediately.

Lemon Buttercream

Makes about		
1 cup (250 mL)		

Use this buttercream to frost Coconut Lemon Moon Cake (variation, page 244) or cupcakes. Leftovers taste good on pancakes.

Tips

Publisher's note: Although raw eggs are considered nourishing in the GAPS diet, they may contain salmonella (see sidebar, page 22). If you prefer to err on the side of caution, use the yolk from a pasteurized in-shell egg, if they are available in your area. Note that, while pasteurized eggs are not part of the GAPS nutritional protocol, food safety must be your first priority.

The buttercream tends to separate a little when stored in the refrigerator for more than 1 day. Remove from refrigerator to let it soften slightly, then just beat it together again.

• ***Electric mixer***

½ cup	butter, softened	125 mL
½ cup	raw honey	125 mL
1	large egg yolk (see tip)	1
	Finely grated zest of 1 lemon	
1 tsp	freshly squeezed lemon juice	5 mL

1. In a bowl, using electric mixer, beat butter and honey until well blended. Beat in egg yolk, lemon zest and lemon juice until thick and fluffy. Use immediately or cover and refrigerate for up to 3 days.

Mocha Buttercream

**Makes about
1 cup (250 mL)**

*When you have progressed
to the point where you
tolerate a nice cup of coffee
made from real beans,
you might also enjoy this
mocha buttercream. It's
great for both frosting and
filling cakes.*

Tips

Publisher's note: Although
raw eggs are considered
nourishing in the GAPS diet,
they may contain salmonella
(see sidebar, page 22). If
you prefer to err on the side
of caution, use the yolk
from a pasteurized in-shell
egg, if they are available in
your area. Note that, while
pasteurized eggs are not
part of the GAPS nutritional
protocol, food safety must be
your first priority.

The buttercream tends to
separate a little when stored
in the refrigerator for more
than 1 day. Remove from
refrigerator to let it soften
slightly, then just beat it
together again.

• *Electric mixer*

½ cup	butter, softened	125 mL
½ cup	raw honey	125 mL
2 tsp	freshly ground coffee	10 mL
1	large egg yolk (see tip)	1
	Finely grated zest of 1 orange	
2 tsp	freshly squeezed orange juice	10 mL

1. In a bowl, using electric mixer, beat butter and honey until well blended. Beat in coffee, egg yolk, orange zest and orange juice until thick and fluffy. Use immediately or cover and refrigerate for up to 3 days.

Vanilla Kefir Cream

Makes 4 servings

What a great way to enjoy probiotic coconut fat! This cream goes well with cakes, fresh fruit, Applesauce (page 219), Apple Jelly with Berries (page 225) and many other desserts.

Tip

In recipes that are not heated, use raw honey for its added health benefits.

- **Electric mixer**

5 tsp	raw honey	25 mL
½	vanilla bean, seeds scraped	½
½ cup	Coconut Kefir (page 93)	125 mL

1. In a bowl, stir honey and vanilla seeds until combined.
2. Using electric mixer, beat in coconut kefir for about 1 minute or until well blended. Use immediately or cover and refrigerate for up to 2 hours.

Variation
Beat in 1 tsp (5 mL) whisky (not smoked) at the end of step 2.

Bourbon Butter

Makes about ½ cup (125 mL)

The delicate flavor of this sauce makes it a perfect topping for muffins (pages 247–249), Christmas Puddings (page 246) or other cakes.

Tip
In recipes that are not heated, use raw honey for its added health benefits.

	Grated zest of ½ orange	
1 tsp	ground ginger	5 mL
6 tbsp	butter, softened	90 mL
2 tbsp	bourbon whiskey	30 mL
4 tsp	raw honey	20 mL

1. In a bowl, mash together orange zest, ginger, butter, whiskey and honey until smooth. Use immediately or cover and refrigerate for up to 1 week. Let soften before using.

Strawberries in Honey

Makes 6 servings

Use this sweet sauce to top pancakes (pages 216–217), waffles (page 218) or Ebelskivers (page 224), along with Sour Cream (page 92) or Coconut Whipped Cream (page 261).

5 oz	frozen strawberries (see tip)	150 g
4 to 5 tsp	raw honey	20 to 25 mL
1/2	vanilla bean, seeds scraped	1/2

1. Quarter berries while frozen, place in a bowl and let thaw.
2. Place honey to taste in a medium bowl and stir in vanilla seeds until combined. Add berries, stirring gently to coat, and let soak until honey has completely dissolved.

Variation

Substitute cherries or raspberries for the strawberries. Adjust the amount of honey according to how sweet or sour the cherries or berries are.

Tips

Fresh strawberries can, of course, be used instead of frozen. Add quartered berries to the honey mixture and let stand until juices are released from the berries.

In place of the vanilla seeds, you can use 1 tsp (5 mL) Vanilla Vodka (page 79) or pure vanilla extract.

Orange Sauce

**Makes about
²/₃ cup (150 mL)**

*Pour this sauce over
Coconut Cake (page 244)
or serve it with pancakes
(pages 216–217) or
Ebelskivers (page 224).*

Tips

In place of the vanilla vodka,
you can use the seeds from
½ split vanilla bean.

This sauce can be stored in
an airtight container in the
refrigerator for up to 1 week.

	Finely grated zest of ½ orange	
6 tbsp	freshly squeezed orange juice (from about 2 oranges)	90 mL
4 tsp	honey	20 mL
1 tbsp	freshly squeezed lime juice (optional)	15 mL
1 tsp	Vanilla Vodka (page 79) or pure vanilla extract	5 mL
2 tbsp	butter	30 mL

1. In a small saucepan, combine orange zest, orange juice, honey, lime juice (if using) and vanilla vodka; bring to a simmer over medium-low heat. Simmer, stirring occasionally, for 10 minutes or until reduced and syrupy.

2. Remove from heat and stir in butter until melted. Let cool for at least 10 minutes or to room temperature.

Holiday Spice Blend

**Makes about
¼ cup (60 mL)**

*This aromatic spice blend
is used to make Mince Tarts
(page 240) and Christmas
Puddings (page 246).*

1 tbsp	ground cinnamon	15 mL
1 tbsp	ground allspice	15 mL
2 tsp	ground nutmeg	10 mL
1 tsp	ground cloves	5 mL
1 tsp	ground coriander	5 mL
1 tsp	ground ginger	5 mL

1. In an airtight container, combine cinnamon, allspice, nutmeg, cloves, coriander and ginger. Use immediately or seal container and store in a cool, dark place for up to 6 months.

Hazelnut Croquant

**Makes enough
for 1 large cake or
4 servings of dessert**

*Nut croquant adds a
wonderful crunch to
a soft cake or dessert.
Use it as garnish or
a hidden surprise.*

Tip

Use this croquant the same
day you make it.

1²⁄₃ oz	dried soaked hazelnuts (see page 74), chopped	50 g
1 tsp	freshly ground coffee (or 1½ tsp/7 mL ground cinnamon)	5 mL
1 tbsp	honey	15 mL

1. In a small dry skillet, toast hazelnuts over medium-low heat, stirring constantly, for about 3 minutes or until fragrant and lightly browned. Immediately transfer to a bowl.

2. Sprinkle coffee (or cinnamon) over nuts and add honey; stir well while honey melts. Pour onto a plate and let cool completely.

3. Scrape nut mixture onto a cutting board and coarsely chop.

Variation

Almond Croquant: Replace the hazelnuts with dried soaked almonds and use 1½ tsp (7 mL) ground cinnamon (not coffee).

Breads

Nut and Seed Bread

Makes 1 loaf

Sometimes it's just nice to have something "bready" to accompany a salad or some cheese, or to eat on its own as a snack.

Tips

This bread crumbles more easily than bread made with flour, so use a sharp serrated knife and, if it starts to crumble when you slice it, try cutting thicker slices.

Wrap cooled bread well and store in the refrigerator for up to 1 week or freeze for up to 3 months.

- **Preheat oven to 325°F (160°C), with rack set in second-lowest position**
- **10- by 4-inch (25 by 10 cm) or 9- by 5-inch (23 by 12.5 cm) glass, stoneware or ceramic loaf pan, greased**

3½ oz	dried soaked almonds (see page 74), coarsely chopped	100 g
3½ oz	dried soaked walnuts, coarsely chopped	100 g
3½ oz	dried soaked pumpkin seeds, coarsely chopped	100 g
3½ oz	dried soaked sunflower seeds, coarsely chopped	100 g
3½ oz	flax seeds	100 g
3½ oz	sesame seeds	100 g
1 tsp	salt	5 mL
5	large eggs	5
⅓ cup	butter, Clarified Butter (page 68) or coconut oil, melted	75 mL

1. In a large bowl, combine almonds, walnuts, pumpkin seeds, sunflower seeds, flax seeds, sesame seeds and salt.

2. In a medium bowl, whisk eggs and butter until well blended. Pour over seed mixture and stir until evenly moistened. Press into prepared loaf pan, smoothing top.

3. Bake in preheated oven for 1 hour or until firm. Transfer loaf to a wire rack and let cool completely.

Variation

You may also choose to make small dinner rolls in muffin pans. Reduce the baking time to 40 minutes.

Banana Bread

Makes 1 loaf

This banana bread is slightly sweet thanks to the ripe bananas and a touch of honey. It goes well with butter or cheese, and a slice makes a nice snack.

Tip

If using vanilla extract, check the label to make sure it contains only vanilla, water and alcohol, with no other additives.

- **Preheat oven to 340°F (170°C), with rack set in second-lowest position**
- **Nut grinder (see box, page 75)**
- **Blender**
- **9- by 5-inch (23 by 12.5 cm) glass, stoneware or ceramic loaf pan, lined with waxed paper and greased with clarified butter**

8 oz	dried soaked almonds (see page 74)	250 g
1 tsp	ground cinnamon	5 mL
Pinch	salt	Pinch
4	large eggs	4
2	ripe bananas	2
3 tbsp	Clarified Butter (page 68)	45 mL
1 tsp	Vanilla Vodka (page 79) or pure vanilla extract	5 mL
1 tsp	honey	5 mL

1. In nut grinder, grind almonds into fine or medium-fine flour.

2. In blender, combine almond flour, cinnamon, salt, eggs, bananas, clarified butter, vanilla vodka and honey; blend until smooth. Spread in prepared loaf pan and smooth top.

3. Bake in preheated oven for about 1 hour or until golden brown. Let cool in pan on a wire rack for 15 minutes, then transfer loaf to rack to cool completely.

Sourdough Starter

Makes about 1 cup (250 mL)

Sourdough starter can be used to make all kinds of breads baked from grain flours, including Rye Bread (page 273) and Whole-Grain Bread (page 274).

Tip

After fermenting, store sourdough starter in the refrigerator in an airtight container. This starter does not require the feeding that is typical for starters. Just store it in the refrigerator and make a new batch when you've used it up. Be sure to start it 48 hours before you plan to bake.

¾ cup	graham or rye flour	175 mL
½ cup	kefir whey (page 94) or yogurt whey (page 92)	125 mL
Pinch	salt	Pinch

1. In a bowl, whisk together flour, whey and salt. Cover and let ferment at room temperature for 48 hours or until it develops a sour aroma and rises and bubbles slightly.

Rye Bread

Makes 3 large loaves

In Denmark, thin slices of this rather hard bread are the base for our famous open-face sandwiches, called smörrebröd. *Rye bread is tasty and filling, and is good with all types of sandwich fillings. This is a large portion: three large loaves. Cut them in half and freeze them until needed.*

Tips

You can knead the dough by hand, but it takes quite a bit of effort! It's much easier to use a stand mixer.

Store cooled bread loosely wrapped at room temperature for up to 1 week (shorter in warm temperatures) or well wrapped in the freezer for up to 6 months. Let thaw, unwrapped, at room temperature. If any mold forms, discard the bread.

Use this recipe as the basis for creating your own rye bread. Experiment with different kinds of flour and kernels. As long as it is a long-rise bread baked with sourdough, it is within the parameters of the GAPS transition diet!

- *Stand mixer, fitted with dough hook*
- *Three 9- by 5-inch (23 by 12.5 cm) glass, stoneware or ceramic loaf pans, very well buttered*

Day 1

1	recipe Sourdough Starter (page 272)	1
5¼ cups	cold water	1.3 L
10 oz	light rye flour	300 g
18 oz	cracked rye kernels	550 g
1 lb	whole wheat flour	500 g
3½ oz	flax seeds	100 g
1⅔ oz	sesame seeds	50 g
1⅔ oz	sunflower seeds or green pumpkin seeds (pepitas)	50 g

Day 2

2 cups + 7 tbsp	cold water	600 mL
2 tbsp	salt	30 mL
1 lb 10 oz	rye flour	800 g

Day 1

1. In mixer bowl, stir together sourdough starter and cold water. Attach bowl to stand mixer with dough hook. Add rye flour, cracked rye, wheat flour, flax seeds, sesame seeds and sunflower seeds; mix on low speed until well incorporated. Cover and let rest at room temperature for 24 hours.

Day 2

2. Add water and salt to dough, stirring well to incorporate. Using the stand mixer on low speed, gradually knead in rye flour; knead for at least 10 minutes or until smooth and elastic.

3. Spoon dough into prepared loaf pans, dividing equally. Cover with a lint-free towel and let rise at room temperature for 6 to 12 hours (or overnight).

4. Preheat oven to 350°F (180°C), with rack set in second-lowest position.

5. Bake for 2 hours or until dark brown on top and loaf sounds hollow when tapped. Remove bread from pans and let cool completely on a wire rack.

Whole-Grain Bread

Makes 1 large loaf

It may take some practice to learn to bake perfect sourdough bread. But once you have the hang of it, you'll never look back. Sourdough bread does take time: it requires hours of slow rising to develop that special taste — and to become gut-friendly.

Tips

Store cooled bread loosely wrapped at room temperature for up to 5 days (shorter in warm temperatures) or well wrapped in the freezer for up to 6 months. Let thaw, unwrapped, at room temperature. If any mold forms, discard the bread.

Be sure to wait to try this recipe until you have followed the GAPS nutritional protocol long enough to recover fully and have had at least 6 months of good health. Introduce it gradually and carefully, keeping in mind that, depending on the severity of your health problem, you may never be able to reintroduce bread into your diet.

- *Stand mixer, fitted with the dough hook*
- *9- by 5-inch (23 by 12.5 cm) glass, stoneware or ceramic loaf pan, very well buttered*

Day 1

1	recipe Sourdough Starter (page 272)	1
2½ cups	water	625 mL
7 oz	graham flour	200 g
7 oz	whole wheat flour	200 g
½ cup	cracked wheat kernels	125 mL
5 tsp	flax seeds	25 mL

Day 2

1 tsp	salt	5 mL
13 oz	whole wheat flour	400 g
	Flax seeds (optional)	

Day 1

1. In mixer bowl, stir together sourdough starter and water. Stir in graham flour, wheat flour, cracked wheat and flax seeds until dough is the consistency of smooth porridge. Cover and let rise in a cool place for 24 hours.

Day 2

2. Stir salt and wheat flour into dough. Using the stand mixer on low speed, knead dough for at least 10 minutes or until smooth and elastic. Cover with a lid and let rise at room temperature overnight.

Day 3

3. Using a silicone spatula, scrape dough into prepared loaf pan. Cover with a lint-free towel and let rise at room temperature for 1 to 3 hours or until 1½ to 2 times the height.

4. Preheat oven to 400°F (200°C), with rack set in second-lowest position.

5. Using a sharp knife, cut a lengthwise slash across bread. Brush bread with water and, if desired, sprinkle with flax seeds.

6. Bake for 1 hour or until dark brown on top and loaf sounds hollow when tapped. Remove bread from pan and let cool completely on a wire rack.

Resources and References

Books and Booklets

Aalborg Funch, Birgit. "P-piller" [Birth control pills]. In *Sund Skepsis* [Healthy skepticism], edited by Lasse Skovgaard. Gjern, Denmark: Forlaget Hovedland, 2006.

Blaser, Martin J. *Missing Microbes: How the Overuse of Antibiotics Is Fueling Our Modern Plagues*. New York: Henry Holt and Company, 2014.

Boberg, Rie. *Olivenolie* [Olive oil]. Copenhagen: Politiken Bøger, 2004.

Campbell-McBride, Natasha. *GAPS Stories: Personal Accounts of Improvement and Recovery through the GAPS Nutritional Protocol*. Cambridge, UK: Medinform Publishing, 2012.

Campbell-McBride, Natasha. *Gut and Psychology Syndrome: Natural Treatment for Autism, ADHD/ADD, Dyslexia, Dyspraxia, Depression and Schizophrenia*, revised ed. Cambridge, UK: Medinform Publishing, 2010.

Campbell-McBride, Natasha. *Put Your Heart in Your Mouth: What Really Causes Heart Disease and What We Can Do to Prevent and Even Reverse It*. Cambridge, UK: Medinform Publishing, 2007.

Danish Technical University. *Helhedssyn på nødder — en risk-benefit vurdering* [A holistic view on nuts — a risk-benefit assessment]. Søborg, Denmark: DTU Fødevareinstituttet, 2015.

David, Elizabeth. *Fransk Landkøkken* [The French country kitchen]. Copenhagen: Hans Reitzel, 1958.

Enig, Mary, and Sally Fallon. *Eat Fat, Lose Fat: The Healthy Alternative to Trans Fats*. New York: Plume, 2005.

Fallon Morrell, Sally, and Kaayla T. Daniel. *Nourishing Broth: An Old-Fashioned Remedy for the Modern World*. New York: Grand Central Life & Style, 2014.

Gottschall, Elaine. *Breaking the Vicious Cycle: Intestinal Health through Diet*. Kirkton Press Ltd, 1994.

Gottschall, Elaine. *Internal Bliss: Recipes Designed for Those Following the Gut and Psychology Syndrome Diet*. Omaha: International Nutrition, 2010.

Grandjean, Philippe. *Only One Chance: How Environmental Pollution Impairs Brain Development — and How to Protect the Brains of the Next Generation*. Oxford University Press, 2013.

Isager, Henrik. *Blinde Pletter* [Blind spots]. Gjern, Denmark: Forlaget Hovedland, 2011.

Lashkov, Baden D. *GAPS Guide: Simple Steps to Heal Bowels, Body and Brain*. Middle River, MD: International Nutrition, 2009.

Lustig, Robert. *Fat Chance: Beating the Odds Against Sugar, Processed Food, Obesity, and Disease*. New York: Plume, 2014.

McGee, Harold. *On Food and Cooking: The Science and Lore of the Kitchen*. London: Hodder and Stoughton, 2004.

Perlmutter, David, with Kristin Loberg. *Brain Maker: The Power of Gut Microbes to Heal and Protect Your Brain — for Life*. London: Hodder & Stoughton, 2015.

Price, Weston A. *Nutrition and Physical Degeneration*, 8th ed. Lemon Grove, CA: Price-Pottenger Nutrition Foundation, 2009.

Ravnskov, Uffe. *Hvorfor et højt kolesteroltal er nyttigt* [Why having a high cholesterol number is advantageous]. Gjern, Denmark: Forlaget Hovedland, 2010.

Ravnskov, Uffe. *Kolesterol, myter og realiteter* [Cholesterol: myths and realities]. Gjern, Denmark: Forlaget Hovedland, 2008.

Taubes, Gary. *Good Calories, Bad Calories: Fats, Carbs, and the Controversial Science of Diet and Health*. New York: Anchor Books, 2007.

Teicholz, Nina. *The Big Fat Surprise: Why Butter, Meat and Cheese Belong in a Healthy Diet.* New York: Simon & Schuster, 2014.

Yudkin, John. *Pure, White and Deadly: How Sugar Is Killing Us and What We Can Do to Stop It.* London: Penguin, 2012.

Articles and Blog Posts

Astrup, Arne. 2014. "A Changing View on SFAs and Dairy: From Enemy to Friend." *American Journal of Clinical Nutrition* 100, no. 6 (December 2014): 1407–8.

Campbell-McBride, Natasha. "One Man's Meat Is Another Man's Poison." *Doctor-Natasha.com* (blog), August 15, 2014. http://www.doctor-natasha.com/one-mans-meat-another-mans-poison.php.

Fallon, Sally. "Ancient Dietary Wisdom for Tomorrow's Children." *The Weston A. Price Foundation for Wise Traditions in Food, Farming and the Healing Arts*, January 1, 2000. http://www.westonaprice.org/health-topics/ancient-dietary-wisdom-for-tomorrows-children/.

Fallon, Sally, and Mary G. Enig. "The Great Con-ola." *The Weston A. Price Foundation for Wise Traditions in Food, Farming and the Healing Arts*, July 28, 2002. http://www.westonaprice.org/health-topics/the-great-con-ola/.

Fallon, Sally, and Mary G. Enig. "Out of Africa: What Dr. Price Dr. Burkitt Discovered in Their Studies of Sub-Saharan Tribes." *The Weston A. Price Foundation for Wise Traditions in Food, Farming and the Healing Arts*, December 1, 1999. http://www.westonaprice.org/health-topics/the-skinny-on-fats/out-of-africa-what-dr-price-dr-burkitt-discovered-in-their-studies-of-sub-saharan-tribes/.

Fallon, Sally, and Mary G. Enig. "The Skinny on Fats." *The Weston A. Price Foundation for Wise Traditions in Food, Farming and the Healing Arts*, January 1, 2000. http://www.westonaprice.org/health-topics/the-skinny-on-fats/.

Hvidman, Lone. "Fødsel ved kejsersnit — en epidemi?" [C-section — an epidemic?] *Tidsskrift for forskning i sygdom og samfund* [Journal for research in disease and society], no. 8 (2008): 103–14.

Le Chatelier, Emmanuelle, Trine Nielsen, Junjie Qin, et al. "Richness of Human Gut Microbiome Correlates with Metabolic Markers." *Nature* 500, no. 7464 (August 29, 2013): 541–46.

Masterjohn, Chris. "Saturated Fat Does a Body Good." *The Weston A. Price Foundation for Wise Traditions in Food, Farming and the Healing Arts*, May 6, 2016. https://www.westonaprice.org/health-topics/abcs-of-nutrition/saturated-fat-body-good/.

Onusic, Sylvia. "Nutrition: The Anti-Aging Factor." *The Weston A. Price Foundation for Wise Traditions in Food, Farming and the Healing Arts*, July 7, 2014. https://www.westonaprice.org/health-topics/abcs-of-nutrition/nutrition-the-anti-aging-factor/.

Sjøgren, Kristian. "Dansk gennembrud: Forskere finder 500 nye tarmbakterier" [Researchers find 500 new intestinal bacteria]. *Videnskab*, July 6, 2014. http://videnskab.dk/krop-sundhed/dansk-gennembrud-forskere-finder-500-nye-tarmbakterier.

Weston A. Price Foundation. "Differences Between the Weston A. Price Foundation Diet and the Paleo Diet." *The Weston A. Price Foundation for Wise Traditions in Food, Farming and the Healing Arts*, October 7, 2013. http://www.westonaprice.org/health-topics/differences-between-the-weston-a-price-foundation-diet-and-the-paleo-diet/.

Podcasts and TV Episodes

Karvandi, Kusha. "Podcast Episode #17: Interview with GAPS Diet author, Dr. Natasha Campbell-McBride," September 12, 2014. https://www.youtube.com/watch?v=dHyI9zlxh8g.

Lustig, Robert. "Fat Chance: Fructose 2.0." *Eating for Health (and Pleasure): The UCSF Guide to Good Nutrition*, UCSF Osher Mini Medical School for the Public, UCTV, October 18, 2013. https://www.youtube.com/watch?v=ceFyF9px20Y.

Peretti, Jacques. *The Men Who Made Us Thin*, episode 3. Directed by Anouk Curry. Aired August 22, 2013, on BBC Two. https://www.bbc.co.uk/programmes/b0392hvt.

Websites

Breaking the Vicious Cycle: www.breakingtheviciouscycle.info

Doctor-Natasha.com: www.doctor-natasha.com

Gut and Psychology Syndrome: www.gaps.me

GAPS Diet: www.gapsdiet.com

The Probiotic Jar: www.theprobioticjar.com

Sugar and Sweetener Guide: www.sugar-and-sweetener-guide.com

Also visit this book's website at www.gapschef.com

Acknowledgments

My warmest thanks to Tressa Lamela, Jenifer Lloyd, Mette Gad and Ole Schröder for their help in the creation of this book; to Inge Lynggaard Hansen and all my supportive friends and family; to the active members of the GAPS groups on Facebook and Yahoo! Helpgroup around the world for their knowledge-sharing and support; to Dr. Irene Hage for the introduction; and to Dr. Natasha Campbell-McBride for so generously sharing her wealth of knowledge on human nutrition and health.

Library and Archives Canada Cataloguing in Publication

Gad, Signe
[GAPS kogebogen. English]
    Using the GAPS diet : 175 recipes for gaining control of your gut flora / Signe Gad ; foreword by Dr. Irene Hage, MD, ND.

Includes index.
Translation of: GAPS kogebogen.
ISBN 978-0-7788-0594-6 (softcover)

    1. Gastrointestinal system—Diseases—Diet therapy. 2. Cookbooks. I. Title.
II. Title: Using the gut and psychology syndrome diet. III. Title: GAPS kogebogen. English.

RC819.D5G3313 2018   616.3'30654   C2018-901854-2

GAPS Diet Index

A
Astrup, Arne, 41

B
bacteria, 14–16. *See also* gut flora
beverages, 204
The Big Fat Surprise (Teicholz), 40–41
bone broth, 23, 27–28, 98

C
Campbell-McBride, Natasha, 11, 14,
    29, 41, 47
Candida albicans, 15
casein intolerance, 90
cheese, 90
cholesterol, 40
coconut, 55
cooking oil, 39

D
dairy products, 90–91
detoxification, 18, 26–27
digestion, 16

E
eggs, 22
Enig, Mary, 41

F
fats, 23, 36–41. *See also* oils
    choosing, 36–39
    monounsaturated, 36, 37
    polyunsaturated, 36
    saturated, 36, 37, 39–41
fiber, 22
fish oil, 39
flours, 55
foods. *See also specific foods*
    allergies to, 42–43
    animal-based, 28
    fermented, 27, 57, 81, 90–91
    intolerance of, 42–43, 90
    organic, 52

    sensitivities to, 21
    shopping for, 52–55

G
GAPS, 14–17
    specialists in, 48–49
    symptoms, 17
GAPS Diet, 18–35
    intro diet, 20–25
    intro diet: meal plans, 58–61
    intro diet: recipes, 24–25
    full diet, 27–32
    full diet: meal plans, 62–63
    full diet: recipes, 30–32
    transition diet, 35
    kitchen equipment, 56–57, 91
    kitchen staples, 68–79
    meal plans, 57–63
    and medications, 44
    purpose, 18–19
    support during, 48–49
    what to avoid, 33–35
    what to eat, 19–35
gelatin powder, 55
gluten intolerance, 43
Good Calories, Bad Calories (Taubes),
    41
grocery shopping, 52–55
Gut and Psychology Syndrome
    (Campbell-McBride), 47
gut flora (microbiome), 11, 14–16, 18

H
healing crisis (Herxheimer reaction),
    26–27
herbs, 29
honey, 29, 54

I
immune system, 15, 47

J
juices, 29, 204

L

lactose intolerance, 42–43
leaky gut syndrome, 16
lifestyle changes, 47

M

meat, 28
    buying, 53, 55
microbes, 14–16. *See also* gut flora
    die-off of, 26–27
milk and cream, 90–91

N

nutrients, 18
nuts, 57

O

oils, 39, 54
olive oil, 37
"One Man's Meat Is Another Man's
    Poison" (Campbell-McBride), 29

P

picky eaters, 44–46
probiotics, 21, 28
Put Your Heart in Your Mouth
    (Campbell-McBride), 41

R

Ravnskov, Uffe, 41

S

seeds, 57
sesame flour, 55
social media, 49
starch, 16
stocks, 23
sugar, 16. *See also* sweeteners
supplements (nutritional), 44
sweeteners, 29. *See also* sugar

T

Taubes, Gary, 41
Teicholz, Nina, 40–41
tomatoes, 54
tomato vinegar, 54

V

vegetable oil, 39
vegetables, 28–29
vinegar, 54

W

water, 54
weight loss, 46–47
whey, 43, 90
*Why Having a High Cholesterol
    Number Is Advantageous*
    (Ravnskov), 41

Recipe Index

A

Aïoli, 188
almonds. *See also* nuts
  blanching, 74
  Almond and Seed Crackers, 200
  Almond Cream, 230
  Almond Tuiles, 252
  Apple or Pear Clafoutis, 234
  Baked Apples, 223
  Banana Bread, 271
  Berry Clafoutis, 235
  Brussels Sprout and Apple Salad, 135
  Cauliflower Couscous, 174
  Cauliflower Gratin, 173
  Christmas Puddings, 246
  Cocoa and Raspberry Muffins, 248
  Cocoa Mousse, 228
  Date and Nut Balls, 258
  Hazelnut Croquant (variation), 267
  Honey Apple Waffles, 218
  Marzipan, 259
  Pear Walnut Muffins, 249
  Rhubarb Crumble, 242
  Salted Almonds, 201
  Tarte Tatin à la GAPS, 238
  Whisky Balls, 257
anchovies
  Beef or Veal Liver Pâté, 126
  Rémoulade, 189
Anise Honey, 78
apple cider
  Apple Jelly with Berries and Coconut Whipped Cream, 225
  Mulled Apple Cider, 213
apples and applesauce
  Apple Cream, 229
  Apple or Pear Clafoutis, 234
  Apple Pork, 154
  Applesauce, 219
  Baked Apples, 223

Brussels Sprout and Apple Salad, 135
Carrot, Apple and Celery Juice, 208
Carrot and Avocado Smoothie, 210
Coconut Cake (variation), 244
Ebelskivers, 224
Fruit Salad Deluxe, 226
Honey Apple Waffles, 218
Mince Tarts, 240
Oven-Baked Mackerel with Apple Compote, 147
Rhubarb Crumble (variation), 242
Spicy Apple Compote, 170
Tarte Tatin à la GAPS, 238
Archipelago Macaroons, 254
asparagus
  Corned Tongue in Mushroom Sauce (variation), 162
  Italian Salad, 133
  White Asparagus with Lemon Butter, 171
avocados
  Carrot and Avocado Smoothie, 210
  GAPS Sushi, 123
  Guacamole, 139
  Lumpfish Roe with Avocado, 122
  Lunch Wraps, 114
  Quick Strawberry Ice Cream, 232

B

bacon
  Beef or Veal Liver Pâté, 126
  Campfire Koftas, 129
  Club Salad, 132
  Fried Liver with Onions and Mushrooms (tip), 159
  Lunch Wraps, 114
  Veal Heart Casserole, 166

bananas
  Banana Bread, 271
  Banana Mazarin Cake, 243
  Banana Pancakes, 216
  Blueberry Muffins, 247
  Carrot and Avocado Smoothie, 210
  Cocoa and Raspberry Muffins, 248
  Cocoa Mousse, 228
  Fruit Salad Deluxe, 226
  Quick Strawberry Ice Cream, 232
  Strawberry Smoothie, 210
beans
  Falafels, 138
  Fish Cakes, 151
  GAPS-Friendly Pizza with a Crispy Crust, 160
  Ginger Pumpkin Pie, 236
  Lunch Wraps (variation), 114
  Mashed Root Vegetables (variation), 181
  Meatballs (variation), 157
  Oven-Baked Vegetables, 180
  Spinach Pie, 178
  White Bean Hummus, 139
  White Beans and Lima Beans, 72
Béarnaise Sauce, 186
beef. *See also* meat; veal
  Beef or Veal Liver Pâté, 126
  Beef Vegetable Soup, 110
  Bolognese Sauce, 158
  Corned Tongue in Mushroom Sauce, 162
beets
  Beet Chips, 198
  Beet Salad, 134
  Mashed Root Vegetables, 181
berries. *See also* fruit, dried
  Apple Jelly with Berries and Coconut Whipped Cream, 225